AIDS
the deadly seed

An anthropological and epidemiological
investigation of a modern epidemic
and its significance

*In memory of
Karl Hugo Zinck*

Translated by Christian von Arnim

RUDOLF STEINER PRESS

Translated by Christian von Arnim from
AIDS — die tödliche Befruchtung : Untersuchungen zur Menschenkunde, Epidemiologie u. Schicksalssprache e. modernen Seuche
© 1988 Verlag Freies Geistesleben GmbH, Stuttgart

Edited by Joan M. Thompson
Cover design by Christiana van Manen

© **Rudolf Steiner Press, Sussex, 1991**

ISBN : 1 85884 130 4

Typeset by Imprint, Crawley Down
Printed and Bound in Great Britain
by Billing and Sons Limited, Worcestershire

Contents

Foreword   5

1. OBJECTIVE THINKING AND
   COMPLEMENTARY KNOWLEDGE   7

   Objective thinking and the structure of scientific consciousness 8 / At the limits of observation 11 / From anatomy to microscopy: 'new' worlds 14 / Dimensional progression: a look at a subsensory world 15 / Complementary knowledge: a methodological requirement 17 / The boundaries of thinking 18 / First steps beyond the frontier — meditation 20 / Cognitive stages in the science of the spirit 21

2. THE HUMAN ORGANISM AND
   ITS CONSTITUENT ELEMENTS   23

   Nutritional methods — cellular and humoural 24 / The construction of the human being through cell-transformation 25 / Stages in the architecture of the organism — stages of cell-deformation 28 / The construction of the human being through the metabolic stream — the external digestion 34 / Humoural circulation: fluid organism-metabolism-protein 35 / Respiration: air organism-rhythm-the fats 37 / Equilibrium: warmth organism-homoeostasis-carbohydrates 38 / Stages of decomposition — releasing the soul element from the body 39 / Natural science — spiritual science. Complementary knowledge 41

3. THE BIOLOGICAL INDIVIDUAL   45

   The threefold structure of the human organism — a key concept 45 / The biological individual 54 / Sexual reproduction — an artifice of nature 57 / Biological self and non-self 57 / Immunology — a biological learning process 58 / The relationship between mental and biological learning 60

4. DIGESTION AND THE IMMUNOLOGICAL
   RECOGNITION OF FOREIGN MATTER   63

   Digestion and the immunological recognition of foreign matter — polar actions of the metabolic system 63 / The blood and the biological individual between dispersion and self-perception 65 / The lymphatic system — an organ of perception in the metabolism 70 / The cellular and humoural instruments of the immunological processes 72 / Processes of specific immunity 73 / Non-specific cellular and humoural immunity 77 / Allergies and inflammation — a polar relationship 80

5. AIDS — THE DEADLY SEED   85

   The new epidemic 85 / Symptomatology of AIDS 86 / AIDS — a venereal disease 91 / The threefold structure and sexual organization 92 / Fertilization — identity of perception and digestion 96 / AIDS — a diseased fertilization 101

6. THE DUAL NATURE OF HUMAN BEINGS.
   AN ESOTERIC EPIDEMIOLOGY
   WITH REFERENCE TO AIDS   107

   Epidemics: are there 'external' demonic forces in nature? 107 / Macro-forms in the realms of nature 111 / The counter-world of the micro-structures 116 / The human being — a dual being 122 / On the origins of demons of illness 126 / An esoteric epidemiology of AIDS 132

7. AIDS — INDIVIDUAL DESTINY AND DISEASE   135

   How the patient feels and medical diagnosis 135 / AIDS — individual destiny and disease 137 / About the destiny of being ill 140 / AIDS — a karmic benefit? 145 / Therapeutic aims — a perspective 147

Foreword

The origin of this study and the relationship between its chapters require a word of explanation. It was not initially my intention to publish the study in book form and it first appeared — with the exception of the last chapter — as a series of six articles in the journal *die Drei*.

The decision to deal with AIDS arose primarily from scientific interest, coupled with an interest in the psychological and social significance for the human race of this new epidemic. Nevertheless, that alone would have been insufficient reason to write about AIDS if I had not also held the view that the systematic study of the human being contained in Rudolf Steiner's Anthroposophy had a decisive and clarifying contribution to make towards an understanding of this illness.

In view of the contribution Anthroposophy can make to an understanding of AIDS, the book begins with material on the methodology of modern micro-biological research and the human being from a medical point of view. These contributions appeared in *die Drei* in October/November 1986. The first contribution, in particular, refers to questions of methodology which concerned me as long ago as the period immediately after the Second World War, when I was a medical student. In this context, conversations with a much-admired friend of mine, Dr Karl Hugo Zinck, who died in 1976, played an important role and I therefore dedicate this study to his memory.

But AIDS also calls for a basic anthroposophical outline of modern immunology and of the individual as a biological entity. The two contributions on this subject appeared in May and June 1987, respectively.

Once the anthropological and medical basis had been established in these essays, the concept of the AIDS disease itself, and its aetiology, could then be developed. This was followed by an outline of an esoteric epidemiology with special reference to AIDS. Both of these appeared in *die Drei* in September/October 1987.

In addition, the book would not have been complete without tracing the development of the illness in individual AIDS patients.

For in this epidemic — quite apart from any aetiological and epidemiological interest — the patient needs to be accompanied in a special and understanding way through the existential crisis which he alone has to face.

Everyone who is aware of the special dimension of this illness will understand that this book does not comment on specific medical treatments. Speculation about remedies divorced from individual cases lacks any foundation. A longer-term perspective of what is necessary to overcome this illness may become clear from the study as a whole.

At first glance this book about AIDS may appear diffuse and lacking in cohesiveness. That is due to its origins, which I have described above. But I am convinced that true medical progress through Anthroposophy can only be achieved if every single phenomenon, every discovery, every symptom is traced back to its fundamental context, to spiritual concepts. Only when they are placed in this larger context do both the individual symptoms as well as the syndrome of AIDS achieve greater illumination. It is more than clear that such illumination is sought today. The psycho-social disturbance provoked by AIDS — oscillating between justified concern and hysteria — demonstrates quite clearly that AIDS must be recognized as an indicator not only of the physical, but also of the psychological and spiritual condition of humanity. It is my desire that this study should make an initial contribution towards penetrating beyond these disturbances in order to gain a clear understanding of their esoteric background and the action which is required.

Wilton
New Hampshire, USA

Klaus Dumke
4th September 1987

CHAPTER ONE

OBJECTIVE THINKING AND COMPLEMENTARY KNOWLEDGE

Current medical and biological knowledge would be inconceivable without the experimental research methods which penetrate into the micro-sphere, and which were first used in the discovery and definition of the cell (Schwann and Schleiden 1838/39). A common thread of research on an increasingly microscopic scale runs from the discovery of that so-called basic building block of plant and animal organisms to the investigation of the micro-structure of cell nuclei, chromosomes and genes, and to the macromolecular structure of these genes and its significance. Today the interest in the visible structure of the organism has been superseded by this invisible micro-world. Biological knowledge deals to a large extent with structures which are not visible as such. Similar progress has been made in the field of physiology — the study of the processes occurring in living organisms. Here, too, research has penetrated into the micro-sphere. As a consequence, life today is conceived of largely in terms of invisible biochemical and bioelectrical micro-processes.

The conventional interpretation of these discoveries cannot be used in anthroposophical anthropology without first examining the methodological foundations of such an interpretation. Furthermore, we have to assess critically its implications for the organism as a whole and, beyond that, for our overall biological and anthropological interpretation of the world.

Objective thinking and the structure of scientific consciousness

We have scientific access to biological structures (organisms or elements thereof) — as to everything else in the world — only through observation and thinking.[1] We accumulate perceptions and then order and classify them conceptually to build up an initially still incomplete but increasingly full image of the nature of such structures or natural processes. We perceive things discretely, our thinking aims for coherence. We can — to choose a simple example — observe and describe the shape of human teeth. The various types of teeth can be ordered conceptually into groups with specific shapes and functions (incisors, canine teeth, molars) and finally into the complete set. Likewise, the individual tooth can only be understood through a combination of perception and conceptualization. Only this can differentiate between crown, neck and root and reassemble these discrete elements into the whole.

Borrowing a term from Goethe, the continuous interaction between perception and thinking, the link between the discontinuous tendencies inherent in perception and the continuity created by thinking might be described as 'objective thinking'.[2] It is a characteristic of ordinary human consciousness in general. Nevertheless, Goethe's concept of 'objective thinking' encompasses more than this ordinary consciousness. We can therefore ask: How does objective thinking arise from the combination of perception and thinking which constitutes our ordinary consciousness?

We use this interaction, the relationship between perception and conceptualization, both statically and dynamically, in both a fixed and a fluid manner. If, for example, we establish that a particular tooth is an incisor, our thinking becomes depictive in character; the general concept 'tooth' is determined and fixed by the concrete content of our perception which shows it to be an incisor. In such a situation we leave out of consideration and ignore

1 Rudolf Steiner, *The Philosophy of Freedom: Philosophy of Spiritual Activity*, Rudolf Steiner Press, London 1988. Chapter Five.
2 J.W. von Goethe, "Bedeutende Fördernis durch ein einziges geistreiches Wort" in *Naturwissenschaftliche Schriften*, Vol. Two, ed. Rudolf Steiner.

the fact that the concept 'tooth' can include a great deal more, i.e. incisor, molar or canine tooth, or the whole set of teeth, or an organ of the digestive system, or an epidermal skeletal organ, and much more. All these connections belong to the total concept of a 'tooth', just as the latter in turn has its place within the organism in the contexts mentioned above. Our depictive thinking excludes all these connections; it *focuses* only on that *particular* incisor which is being observed at that moment.

Our commonplace perceptual thinking is characterized by attaching itself to an idea in this way.[3] Yet in life we have to progress from one percept to the next, that is, from one idea to another. In doing so, we are very often not fully aware of the links which lead from one to the other — our everyday consciousness proceeds by focusing on a discontinuous and disjointed chain of ideas.

By contrast, Goethe's objective thinking takes fixed concepts and expands them as the content of perception changes. In this way a given perceptual structure, an incisor for example, becomes the point of departure for a wealth of overlapping relationships developing in very different directions. Our thinking expands and becomes more flexible. On the other hand, if we strengthen the intensity of our observation, the perception and idea of an 'incisor' forms the basis on which to look even more closely at, and differentiate between, single elements such as crown, neck, root, defective enamel, receding gums, etc., and thus sub-divide the concept even further.

With objective thinking, the scientist is moving in a field which in principle is infinitely wide and he moves between the poles of unbroken differentiation and combination without ever standing still in one spot, i.e. without becoming fixed. Nevertheless, the fluid interaction of these active cognitive tools is not an arbitrary one. The conceptual context provokes questions which can only be answered with the help of observation. (Here we might recall Goethe's discovery of the intermaxillary bone as the result of wider ideas he was pursuing.) Conversely, every observation leads to a wealth of questions which can only be answered by the thinking it provokes. Our

---

3   Rudolf Steiner, *The Philosophy of Freedom*, Chapter Six.

observation, which tends towards singularity, and our thinking, which establishes relationships, move in opposite directions in objective thinking, but they do so in continuous reciprocal rapport with one another. That is how structure is created in the field of consciousness which stretches between these two elements;[4] observation and thinking interweave like warp and weft and construct what can be called a systematic view of existence. Such a scientific world view is created through our cognitive action to become the 'fabric of reality', that is, a tapestry of warp and weft, of observation and thinking.

This view of the world must be seen as a hierarchical structure. The example of the tooth can demonstrate this once again. We can progress from the individual tooth to the set of teeth; for that we need our thinking. If we used nothing but our observation we would perceive only tooth, tooth, tooth... Through our thinking we take the step from tooth to set of teeth, with the latter being of a higher order. Conversely, we can descend from the tooth to crown, neck and root, for which we make use of our differentiating observation. If we remained with the fixed concept of a tooth all these various structures would elude us.

This systematic world view is more than just an interlaced structure; it comprises sub-divisions and greater unities which in principle are unlimited. In other words, its architecture is hierarchical. Observation and thinking interact wherever we begin to activate our cognition within this architecture. We, the researchers, not the object or the biological structure, decide whether we wish to move in a conceptual or a perceptual direction. Therefore such an object or structure cannot help us determine whether it is a concept or a percept. On the contrary, it always comprises both. Isolated detail and global context interpenetrate one another within it. Every object, every biological structure, indeed, every structure in the world, is a 'tapestry' in the above sense, the action of global forces grasped by observation and thinking.

All this leads to the conclusion that scientific consciousness requires particular care in order not to distort the reality it constructs. Scientists have to muster the courage to pursue one-sidedly either

---

[4] Herbert Witzenmann, *Strukturphänomenologie*, Dornach 1983.

the path of observation or of conceptualization, sometimes to a considerable degree. Without this courage we would be left with nothing but frozen depictions of ideas. Nevertheless, our conceptual and perceptual forays must lead to balance, notwithstanding their flexibility. And indeed, such one-sided forays of thinking and observation will correct themselves if balance is part of our scientific aims.[5] It is precisely the achievement of balance between these two arms of scientific investigation, while still extending their reach, which characterizes Goethe as a scientist, and also as a master of objective thinking.

At the limits of observation

We are now in a position to enquire whether our consciousness, with its systematic network of observation and thinking, is limited in any way, whether there are any barriers to observation and thinking. Indeed, there are, and we can experience those barriers in a number of ways. Our observation is limited at two levels:

1. Organisms, particularly animal and human ones, offer themselves to observation from the outside. The interior of the body below the surface of the skin is not accessible to the eye; the interior structure is hidden. We can only gain access and see what is going on through surgical *intervention* which breaks through and progresses beyond the normal observational limits. It does so by means of the experimental modification of the organism. Ordinary observation within objective consciousness does not need such intervention: in a certain sense the intervention only affects the researcher, and only in this sense can the research be described as experimental. A biologist who wants to observe the effect of the sunrise on a blossom at five o'clock in the morning, or something similar, has to make sure he arrives at that particular place at the given hour. The plant itself is not affected by his action. If we leave

---

5 J.W. Goethe, "Der Versuch als Vermittler von Objekt und Subjekt", in *Naturwissenschaftliche Schriften*, Vol. Two.

aside operations, endoscopies and vivisection, anatomical intervention can only be carried out on corpses. It destroys the natural cohesion of the organism. Death is the precondition. The latter in itself is already an intervention in the organism, in that it is the natural method by which the cohesion of the organism's various elements — which we call life — is dissolved. The anatomical and histological intervention carried out by scientists therefore only continues what has begun with death. They merely do it by different methods and with different equipment from that of natural decomposition. Consequently, anatomical intervention has two effects: it dissolves the given structure and in doing so discloses to the eye of the observer a wealth of new, as yet unknown, information which remains hidden to the non-experimental observer. Anatomy as dissection begins at *the boundary of life and death,* that is to say, at the boundary where the naturally observable outer organism ends and the experimentally disclosed inner organism begins.

2. But this process of dissection, taken one step further, itself comes up against another boundary: the boundary of the micro-sphere. This boundary to the *micro-sphere* arises where our sense organs — primarily the eye — are no longer able to perceive a difference, a discontinuity in a given structure — a section of tissue, for example. This is referred to as the resolving power of the sensory organs which have reached their limit here. We know that this limit is reached with the eye when the impression on the retina only affects one cell of the retina. If a structure is big enough for its optical image to affect two directly adjacent vision cells of the retina, that structure is still differentiated from its surroundings. The boundary of the resolving power therefore approximately coincides with the dimension of the cell.

The observational side of objective thinking, then, extends to this boundary. All micro-research, the results of which — as we noted earlier — comprise by far the largest part of biological and medical thinking today, is based on extending the reach of anatomical and microscopic observation through the use of instruments; through the artificial lengthening of the extent of our observation. The study of anatomy revealed things hidden to non-experimental research; microscopy — without going into the technical details here —

opens a further world of detail, of differentiation to the observer, where the naked eye makes no distinction. Here, too, the discovery of a wealth of new, so far unknown, findings is connected with the dissolution, indeed, the destruction of the organic growth of the whole. But the balance between whole and part, between thinking and observation, is thereby distorted through the extensive, hypertrophied perceptual element and the reduced conceptual element. [6]

That is the reason why we must ask at this second boundary whether beyond this limit the researcher can continue to relate thinking and observation to each other in the sense of objective thinking, as he did before. In other words, is our usual way of thinking, including the objective thinking of someone using the Goethean method, still valid in any way when it relates to a wealth of perceptions in areas of nature which are made accessible purely experimentally, i.e. by secondary means?

This question is rarely ever asked. On the contrary, scientific research since Schwann and Schleiden has been conducted in a manner which continues to use depictive thinking in a naive and uncritical manner even when it goes beyond the limits of normal observation. Occasionally we also find that the boundary is crossed in this uncritical manner in studies based on Goethean method which have dealt with micro-structures — in spite of Goethe's warning that he felt strangely uncomfortable where microscopes, telescopes and even glasses were concerned.

In order to throw some light on this discomfort, it is my intention to pursue the question systematically and critically because it is of decisive importance for an anthroposophically-based anthropology and biology if we wish to make an anthroposophical contribution to orthodox biology and medicine. This question also plays an important role in a purely orthodox scientific approach to research; only if the answer accords with reality can such research be guided in a healthy direction — as far as the scientific view of the world, and thus any medical practise, is concerned — in interpreting the results of its observation.

[6] Analogously, instrumental telescopy has a similarly distorting effect in astronomical research. It therefore also requires critical examination along the lines being suggested here.

But before we deal with this question directly, let us briefly consider the material made available through anatomy and microscopy.

From anatomy to microscopy: 'new' worlds

Human beings, when they are alive, present objective thinking with a direct sensory and supersensory impression of what they are through their shape, form, expression, gestures, upright posture and much else. In this sense the directly visible impression made by human beings is of an expressive nature. They are 'pictures' [7]. The corpse, deprived of life, of language as an expression of the soul, of its uprightness and movement as an expression of the 'I', still retains some formal if rigidified vestiges of what was present before death. Once the anatomist takes over, structures begin to emerge which are *less and less an expression* of the nature of the human being as a whole, living, ensouled personality.

In the first instance, the anatomist encounters *systems*: bone structure and muscular system, nervous system and blood circulation. These systems still retain something of the characteristics of the whole human being because they penetrate man as a whole, and we can still recognize the latter in outline, even if in an extremely one-sided form. The skin as a systemic organ and — even less apparent — the system comprising the gastro-intestinal tract also maintain vestiges of the complete image of the human being.

Next, the anatomist encounters *organs*. These — for example the liver, kidneys, spleen, lungs, etc. — no longer display any of the characteristics of the human being as a whole. We enter a foreign and in some ways disconcerting world. The organs, in contrast to the systems, are located topographically. The relationship between systems and organs is fluid in so far as the latter may be incorporated in the former: the brain in the nervous system, the heart in the circulatory system, and so on.

---

7   Rudolf Steiner, *Anthroposophical Leading Thoughts*, Rudolf Steiner Press, London 1985, letter of 18 May 1924: 'On the picture-nature of man'.

Just as the systems and organs are subdivisions of the total organism, so the organs in turn are hierarchically subdivided into functional units. These are multi-cell structures which make up the organ in homologous duplication: the hepatic lobule in the liver, nephron in the kidney, pulmonary lobule in the lungs, etc.

Finally, the *cell*, which occurs in the total organism in various forms, structures and sizes, represents the last sub-organization which is visible. It is mostly between the organs and their functional units that we find the second boundary described earlier, at which our observational capacity needs to be reinforced: the advance into the micro-sphere beyond the resolving power of the eye. There are only a few cells in the organism which can be seen with the naked eye; the female egg cell, for example (ca. 200 µ = 0.2 mm diameter).

The dimension of the cell in turn represents a decisive threshold. We can define and identify its components with the microscope in great detail today, but the organism itself in its living context does not breach this boundary — it develops upwards, using the single cell as its starting point. The dimension of the cell therefore represents the micro-boundary of human life. In order to avoid complicating the issue, we cannot here go into a corresponding classification of the even smaller-scale units which are to be found below cell size.

Dimensional progression: a look at a subsensory world

If we look back at the progression from the anatomy as a whole to the histological and cytological levels, the following conclusion presents itself: at each stage a new sub-organization is uncovered as the larger context is broken down. We descend in stages of dimension from the organism as a whole through the systems to organ level, then from the organs to their functional units and, finally, to cell level. In this process of reduction the organism 'breaks down' into a number of systems, several organs, innumerable functional units and, finally, into a myriad of cells. At each stage there is a reduction in the individual characteristics of each component. The cell — with a great deal of variation in form and structure — nevertheless only repeats an elemental basic pattern: nucleus and nuclear membrane, cytoplasm and cell membrane.

Thus experimental observation, assisted by anatomical study and the microscope, reveals a perspective which starts in the foreground with the complete human being and finishes up with the cell (see Diagram 1).

Diagram 1

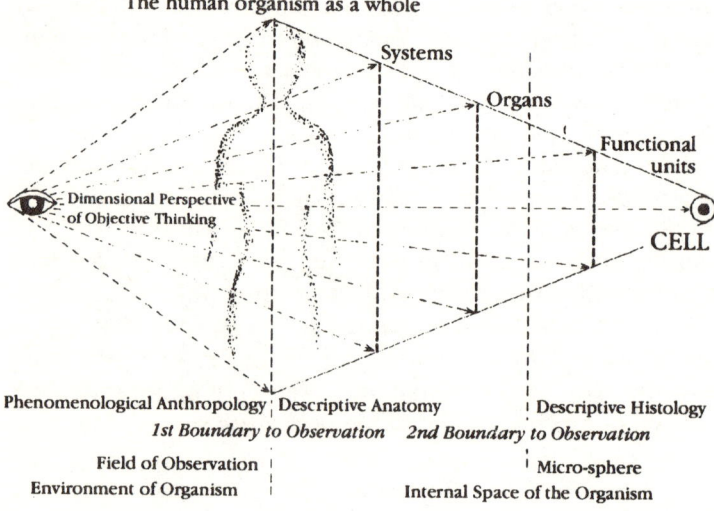

The perspective of the organism sketched out above enables us to define more precisely our earlier critical question: Are the perceptual elements uncovered by the reduction, and, indeed, the destruction of unity, real forms? Are they phenomena in the sense that they are true manifestations of a reality?

On the basis of the ideas we developed earlier, the answer must be no. Because reality is created only by the balanced interaction of observation and thinking. But here we are dealing with the one-sided augmentation of observation and the simultaneous destruction of any unifying elements — in other words, the absence of thinking. Only uncritical force of habit allows our judgement to proceed from the sphere of objective thinking into an area beyond the natural boundaries of the observable world of the senses.[8] Such judgement is no longer valid beyond these boundaries, yet the assumption is always made that it is. Systems, organs and cells are not independent entities of a biological nature. Their appearance is not a phenomenon in a phenomenological sense, because they lack the concepts which define the organism as a whole, concepts which need to be developed to penetrate them with the thinking. On the contrary, they are artefacts disclosed by secondary means, elements in a world beyond the sensory world, the world which can be experienced with the senses. They are, in a certain sense, elements of a 'subsensory world'.[9]

Complementary knowledge: a methodological requirement

We now need to ask the question: How can we reach *reality* from this subsensory world? How can we reach a reality which is consistent with the discovery of these artefacts in a way which makes it possible to integrate them into the larger context, which guides us back from one-sided intensified observation to reality as a totality? Are there ways of creating by other means an awareness of the forces of integration which have been eliminated by the advance of experimental, and thereby destructive, observation? Can the more intense use of the thinking part of our consciousness re-establish the balance in our cognition?

These questions indicate that a *complementary knowledge* is required. The extension of the observational side into the inner and micro-structures of organisms brings both profit and loss: profit through the exposure of elements which we would not otherwise know about; loss through the reduction of reality to artefacts. The extension of observation must be complemented by the extension of thinking, and reality must be restored

---

8   Rudolf Steiner, *The Boundaries of Natural Science*, Anthroposophic Press, New York 1982.
9   Rudolf Steiner, *Anthroposophical Leading Thoughts*, Letter of 12 April 1925: 'From Nature to Sub-Nature'.

through such complementary knowledge. It may be assumed from the circumstances which we have discussed that this reality will be of a higher order than the one effective in the area to which objective thinking applies.

As supersensory knowledge, the science of the spirit, or Anthroposophy, crosses the boundary of objective consciousness in an 'upwards' direction, that is to say, into the supersensory sphere, in the same way as natural science has crossed the boundary of observation into the subsensory sphere, as described earlier. It is therefore a legitimate source for the *complementary knowledge* (called for above) which is needed to integrate the discoveries of natural science which are devoid of reality. We must examine whether we can succeed in restoring reality by utilizing the findings of Anthroposophy about the supersensory part of the human being.

The boundaries of thinking

Having looked at the boundaries of observation and beyond, we have now reached the stage where it is necessary for us to turn our sights towards the boundaries of what we experience as thinking. Within the framework of this study it is not possible to investigate in every detail all the significant aspects of thinking as it reaches its boundaries. We have to restrict ourselves to a brief survey. The boundary which a person encounters in his thinking is not as evident as the one encountered in observation. It is even less evident to the naive consciousness. Historically, the awareness of the natural boundaries of sensory perception arose with the modern age — simultaneously with the wish to break through these boundaries experimentally. The spiritual configuration of the twentieth century, however, contains both the willingness and the awakening ability to pay increasingly greater attention to the boundaries of consciousness with respect to our thinking. Nevertheless, a *change in perspective* is required!

The fundamental approach of objectively-orientated thinking as it creates order out of the multitude of perceptual elements is a naive one. However, this approach leads to an almost complete lack of awareness of the real nature of thinking itself. Precisely because thinking actively immerses itself *in* 'things', the objects, the entities which make up the perceptible world, its view of one unique 'object', the process of thinking itself, is obscured. That is why a change of perspective is required to reflect on the essence of thinking if we want to find the boundary we are seeking. This change in perspective introduces an 'exceptional state' in our normal consciousness. The new perspective can be formulated within our normal naive, object-bound mode of thinking as a new question: How does thinking, which we use unquestioningly all the time, arise? Can we perceive something which would otherwise remain concealed — the perception of thinking as a process *sui generis*?

In pursuit of this question, which alters our conceptual perspective, we reach the boundary we are seeking. What form does the latter take? Initially, thinking displays its content. The conceptual content itself — extensive in nature in contrast to the singularity of perception — is the boundary we encounter, just as our perceptions encounter their boundaries. The conceptual network which spreads out before our mental gaze is potentially all-embracing, encompassing all that is contained in the world, even if that view only ever comprises one — self-chosen — segment. Our mental gaze is captured by the conceptual content of our thinking so that it becomes incapable of penetrating these universally extending relationships in a direction which would give it access to the underlying origins of the thought process. As a result, the thinker's attention generally returns from this boundary — saturated by the conceptual content — to the field of objective consciousness where it seeks to mingle with the elements of perception.

However, if we remain in the exceptional state induced by this new perspective on thinking — thinking which becomes the object of its own cognition — we can gain some significant fundamental understanding at the frontier to the spirit:

1. Thinking is not given without me — unlike sense perceptions. It has to be produced by me. Its universal nature is tied to my individuality. Its content only appears in the consciousness through *thinking action*.

2. Although thinking can only occur through me, the *relationship of thoughts* to one another is an independent, self-supporting and universal structure of ideas. Because one thought supports another, the result is a consistent, equally extensive and intensive, infinite cosmos of thoughts.

3. The paradox between the first and second of these fundamental experiences can only be resolved if our advance towards the origins of thinking uncovers the deeper connection between these two apparently mutually exclusive statements. The separation of the individual elements of perception on the one hand and the universal conceptual relationships on the other, which is possible with everything else, is not possible here. Thinking is an indivisible threefold unity. Thinking in which the individuality of the thinker does not become fully a part of the universal context of his concepts and, equally, thinking which does not fully individualize the idea, is not *true thinking*. That is the basis for the uniqueness of thinking: it unites concept and percept through the action of the *self*. Therefore thinking is not an object, like everything else in the world, but a *fact* — the fundamental fact of the human spirit. [10]

First steps beyond the frontier — meditation

These fundamental experiences of the human spirit presuppose certain requirements: the experimental advance beyond the boundaries of naive thinking into a field of experience which is hidden from objective consciousness. Anthroposophy describes the methodology for such an advance as meditation. Thus meditation is the experimental cognitive advance up to and beyond the frontiers of objective consciousness. Meditation crosses these frontiers with regard to thinking in the same way that objective consciousness uses methods of instrumental observation to cross the frontiers of perception. The anatomist looks through the microscope and thereby gains access to a new world beyond the

---

[10] Rudolf Steiner, *The Philosophy of Freedom*, Chapter Three.

boundaries of natural observation. The researcher in the science of the spirit prepares his thinking through the purely soul-spiritual process of meditation to be the instrument with which he can look into the supersensory world.

In accordance with the three experiential steps described above, meditation posits three conditions which have to be fulfilled in order that we can begin to experience crossing the frontier:

1. Our thinking must concentrate on a thought or image which remains the same for the duration of the meditation. This halts the motion from one subject to the next which takes place in ordinary thinking. This arrest of the thought process leads to an intensification of the way in which thinking experiences itself.

2. In choosing a relevant subject for meditation, the attention is guided into a purely spiritual context which in itself is devoid of perceptual elements. Such subjects are symbolic thoughts, either as a sequence of words or, alternatively, as an image. This enables the meditating person to maintain a free, symbolically structured context for his thinking which is not tied to any sensory perception.

3. Meditation leads to purely inner breathing. For the motion of the spirit in the process of meditation oscillates between experience of the self in the awareness of our thinking intention, and experience of the world as it relates to the content of the meditation.

Although these three conditions, which are simultaneously meditative experiences, can be described separately, they all come together in proper meditation. The threefold unity of thinking which was mentioned earlier becomes a concrete meditative experience.

Cognitive stages in the science of the spirit

The anthroposophical science of the spirit develops through the systematic enhancement of spiritual experiences as it progresses towards and beyond the boundaries of thinking, described above. It continues in the development of the three fundamental meditative experiences by means of esoteric schooling. It reports its findings on three supersensory levels called Imagination, Inspiration and Intuition. We can do no more than mention them here and refer to the relevant literature. [11]

Human beings learn more about the spiritual world at each of these three stages of knowledge. Human beings originate in these spiritual realms and in descending from the spiritual world they bring with them an element of their being from each stage as they assume their physical form in the sensory world. The succession of these elements will be developed in the next chapter in so far as this is relevant in complementing medical diagnosis.

---

11   Rudolf Steiner, *Theosophy*, Rudolf Steiner Press, London 1989; *Knowledge of the Higher Worlds. How is it achieved?*, Rudolf Steiner Press, London 1976; *Occult Science. An Outline*, Rudolf Steiner Press, London 1979.

CHAPTER TWO

THE HUMAN ORGANISM AND ITS CONSTITUENT ELEMENTS

The human being is essentially a spiritual being — an 'I'. In order for human beings to incarnate on a physical-sensory level, they require a structure for the 'I' which allows this spiritual being to become active in the body. Their soul element is active as soul structure or astral body. Such a soul structure also organizes the soul elements of animals into their bodies. The life processes are similarly organized: The plant has its etheric body, while human beings have their own specifically human etheric bodies. In order to exist on earth on a physical-sensory level, human beings additionally require a physical body as that element which provides the supersensory basis for the spatial structure of the organism.[12]

These four structural elements should be thought of as integrated supersensory fields of activity. They are directly perceptible to spiritual research on a supersensory level; objective consciousness can use them as convenient categories.[13] These elements combine to form the human structure as a totality. The ego-organization is in overall control in human beings, the astral body in animals, the etheric body in plants; each element is subordinated to the preceding one, giving a hierarchical structure (Diagram 2, page 24). It should be noted that the human 'I' penetrates through the astral and etheric bodies into the physical body, as do each of the other elements through their subordinate ones. Human beings do not possess animal astral bodies or plant etheric bodies; all the elements are purely human.

12 Rudolf Steiner, *Theosophy*, Chapter One: 'The Nature of Man'.
13 Rudolf Steiner, *Occult Science. An Outline*, Chapter One: 'The Character of Occult Science'.

Diagram 2

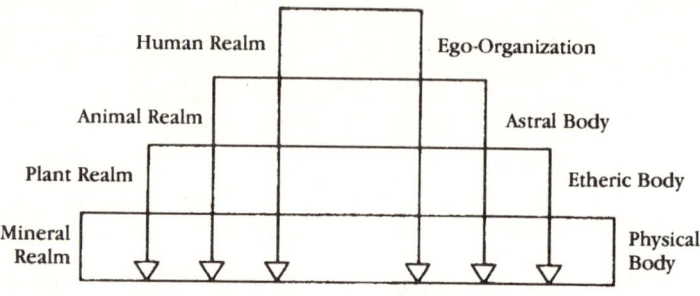

Nutritional methods — cellular and humoural

However, human beings as outlined would be invisible if this structured, supersensory entity did not make itself visible through the absorption of material substance. This absorption takes place in two ways:

1. The first substance which supersensory human beings absorb is the fertilized egg cell. It represents a kind of primary or archetypal nourishment. It has the characteristics of a cell; i.e. not some kind of amorphous nutritional substance, but formed life contained in the body of the cell. The egg cell is fertilized to put it into the state which must be assumed by all nutrition, namely an undifferentiated state. Among the purposes of fertilization is that of 'creating chaos'[14] in the structured protein of the egg cell so that it is put into an undifferentiated state. This state is necessary if the elements which make up the human being are to penetrate and absorb the 'cellular nutrition'.

2. The second method of nutrition occurs across the placenta after the membranes surrounding the embryo have begun to function. Following birth, nourishment is no longer provided through the umbilical cord but comes externally through the gastro-intestinal tract. This nourishment is humoural in character.

---

14 Rudolf Steiner, *World History in the Light of Anthroposophy*, Rudolf Steiner Press, London 1977, lecture of 30 December 1923.

Here the substance providing nourishment is not in the form of cell structures but enters the organism in formless, semi-liquid consistency. Below, we will consider further that the stage of undifferentiation, of chaos, must be passed through at this point as well. The supersensory human being makes consecutive use of two different streams of substance to build himself up:
  a) the hereditary stream — a stream of cellular substance;
  b) the nutritional stream — a stream of humoural substance.

We will see that these two streams are present in human beings throughout their development.

The construction of the human being through cell-transformation

Let us begin by considering the stream of cellular construction. The occurrence which starts with the fertilized egg and ends with birth can be described in four stages, which are determined by the different constituent elements of the human organism and similarly interpenetrate one another:

The *physical element* has the task of restricting life within spatial limits. In this respect the cell as such is an expression of the physical principle. Cell division as a formative principle — which occurs throughout life, starting with the egg and ending with the death of the fully grown organism — is an expression of the physical principle in the sense that space is occupied. Life as a pure process unconnected with space is placed in a spatial setting through this principle. If this principle were active on its own, the cells would all separate to fill space individually. In the closed metazoic, i.e. multi-celled, organism this principle works exclusively only in two instances. First, with cell death in which the dying cell is detached from its cluster and expelled; second, with reproductive cells which detach themselves alive from the cluster in which they are formed.

The latter process demonstrates that human reproductive cells approach ever closer to the physical principle. This orientation — of total detachment from life — reaches its climax with fertilization: here the cell becomes undifferentiated physical 'nourishment' for the supersensory human being, as we noted earlier.

The *etheric element* works to counter the physical principle. It takes hold of the cell material and overcomes the separating, excluding principle by incorporating and embedding the cells in a larger structure. By this means tissue is formed which transcends the cell. Here the separating principle of the physical, and the unifying principle of the etheric, interpenetrate most closely.

If we observe in cell division that there is a continuous repetition of the same, we are looking at the etheric, the life principle; we are describing one of the ways in which life manifests itself. If we look at the separation, the spatial structuring of life which is manifest in the cells, we are describing the physical principle. What we call tissue therefore shows, in contrast to the individual cell, the predominance of the etheric in the organism. In tissue, the formation of cell-transcending structures is recurring: the repetitive principle of the etheric body is dominant.

This polar interaction in tissues between physical and etheric tendencies can be seen as something which we can describe as cell-transformation, and is analogous to the metabolism, which we will discuss later. Each time cell division takes place within living tissue, the pendulum swings towards the physical side at that spot. But the subsequent integration of the two daughter-cells into the tissue allows the etheric principle to recapture the lead and regain the upper hand. Cell-transformation in tissues represents a continuous motion which is subordinated to the unchanging state of the tissue as a whole, the organ. The current of cell-transformation gives expression to the etheric body on the level of cellular substance.

Now tissue does not exist *in abstracto* but always in the context of particular organs and in a particular location. That gives it specific characteristics. This occurs through the action of the *astral element*. The latter is completely different in its form of expression from the etheric body but both of them interact closely. The internal structures of the organism, which provide the basis for all the organs, have their origin in the astral body. This process can be observed most clearly in the formation of the lung during the embryonic stage: there is a bud in the upper digestive tube which turns in on itself, and this inclination to turn in on itself converges with the area of tissue-formation — the raw material, as it were — created by the etheric body. In principle, this process is the same for all the internal organs, although there is a great deal of variation.

By extension we can say, therefore, that all the internal organs are — like the lung — 'respiratory organs', by which we mean the process itself and not the specific inhalation and exhalation of air by the lung.

Whereas the fundamental expression of the physical body is division and thus expansion into space, the astral body has the fundamental organic expression of breathing or, more generally, the rhythmical interchange between inside and out. In between the two, the etheric body is characterized by the endless repetition of the same. The principle of the internal structures as an expression of the astral body can be seen in the functional units, i.e. the characteristic building blocks of the organs, in the same way as they also demonstrate the tendency towards the millionfold repetition of the same structure as an expression of the etheric body.

The 'I' unites these elements through its dominant presence so as to produce a complete and unified human structure in visible form, i.e. with the characteristic human shape. This shows us that ego-organization is responsible for the entire self-contained, outwardly visible form. The three subordinate elements of the human being do not reach the end stage of their development. On the way there, higher principles take hold of them and restrict them in their specific formative tendencies.[15] That is why we do not find in the human being the presence of minerals, plants or animals which exist in nature, even though all these stages are incorporated in the human organism. They are merely hinted at — their form controlled by the ego-organization. That, incidentally, is where the roots of the scientific controversy about the law of recapitulation (also called the law of biogenesis) can be found. At no stage in their development from the egg onwards are human beings effectively animal; but their growth includes developmental principles which, when allowed to run their full course, result in visible animal forms because they have not been restricted in their development by the ego. If the law of recapitulation is understood in this sense, namely as an expression that the four realms of nature are present in the

15 Rudolf Steiner and Ita Wegman, *The Fundamentals of Therapy*, Rudolf Steiner Press, London 1983, Chapter Five.

human being but do not develop into separate identities, then it may be taken as valid. It then becomes an expression of the far-reaching, subordinating relationship between the human being and the realms of nature.

The dominance of the 'I', which we have referred to several times, should be understood as a principle which penetrates all structures and subdivisions. Every single cell in the organism — if healthy — must be seen within its field of activity. This can also be demonstrated experimentally. It has been shown that cells belong to specific organisms, i.e. to structures organized by a particular 'I'.[16] Thus, while the 'I' stamps its individuality on the whole organism, including cells, the variation among cells, their great differentiation according to which organs and tissues they inhabit, arises primarily because of the wealth of formative impulses which the astral body injects into the organism. The astral body therefore does not tend towards the repetition of the same — as the etheric body does — but, on the contrary, towards the modification and alteration of the various shapes. In other words, metamorphosis in seamless stages.

Stages in the architecture of the organism — stages in cell-deformation

Since we cannot here develop the subjects of embryology or histology, we will at least attempt to outline three stages in the gradual increase in cell-deformation which occurs through the action of the supersensory elements in the human being:

We observed that the etheric body integrates the individual cell into the larger tissue formation. The structuring principle of the physical body (cell division) and the linking principle of the etheric body (cell clusters) work together to form biological tissue through the repetition of the same cell type. The action of the astral body in turn integrates the different tissues into specific organs or organ-like structures. Here organ-specific cell

---

16 Hartwig Cleve, 'Die genetisch determinierte biochemische Individualität', in: *Therapiewoche* 41/1985, pp.4694 — 4699.

differentiation takes place in which a degree of deformation can be shown to occur.

This deformation is comparatively slight in the large glandular metabolic organs — the centres of vitality in the organism. Here we still encounter a relative proximity to the early embryonic cell forms. These cells act with youthful vitality. The formative impulse of the astral body, that is to say, of the organ-building principle, does not yet affect the cell itself very deeply. It brings about the specific shape which the tissue is meant to assume through an ordering of the cells from the outside, as it were. This might be described as an *additive formative principle*. The specific histological structure is brought about by ordering the cells like building bricks. The etheric body finds expression in the infinite multiplication of these 'building bricks' as the source for organic 'repetition of the same', while the astral body is expressed in the formation of hollows as the creator of organic internal space. Etheric body and astral body interact very closely in these metabolic organs. Thus the functional units with glandular duct-like structures originate in the intestine and the pancreas, and, in transformation, in the liver and the kidneys (see Illustration 1, below).

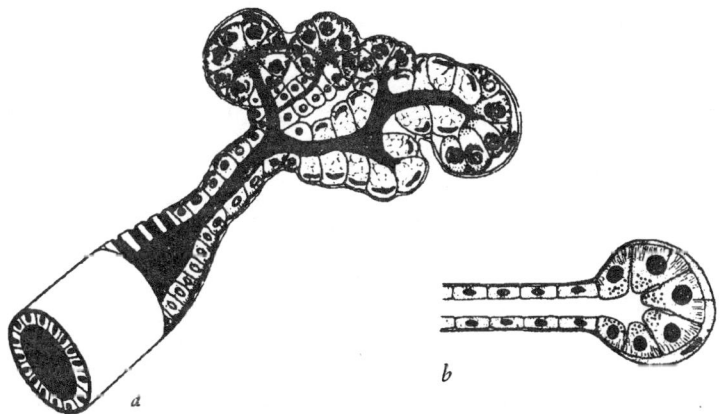

Illus. 1a: Seromucous gland as an example of additive construction.
Illus. 1b: Glandular endpiece (From: Rohen/Lütjen-Drecoll, *Funktionelle Histologie*, Schattauer, Stuttgart/New York 1982).

If we progress to the next, higher stage of histological structures, an increase in deformation takes place. A new formative principle is at work. Here the structure of the tissue is not created by the addition of cells but through the ordering and structuring of substances which, because they exist outside the cell, are described as extracellular substances (see Illustration 2a). Here a higher formative principle is at work, which allows the creation of structures of much greater complexity than the 'additive' method. The cell-deformation which takes effect here leads to the cell substance being 'squeezed out'. The cell secretes a substance which is no longer tied to the cell, the so-called ground substance. This material, mostly of a gel-like or of a fibrous nature, can now serve the astral body more intensely. We might describe this construction method as *plastic-synthetic*, in contrast to additive, because, instead of building bricks, a supra-cellular building material without a prescribed form is being used. These processes lead to much greater

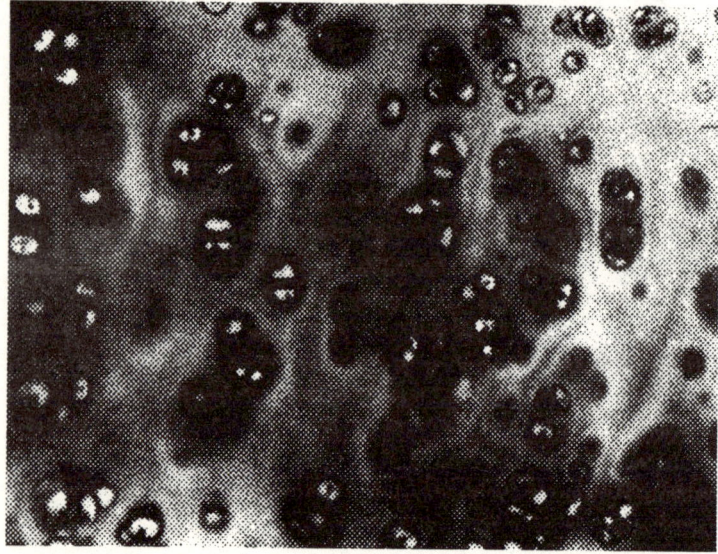

Illus. 2a: Hyaline cartilage tissue as an example of plastic-synthetic construction. The cartilage cells can be seen embedded in their ground substance.

penetrative interlacing among the deformed cells. What appears as deformation in the cell, signifies for the organism as a whole the next, higher stage in its construction, brought about by the more intense action of the astral body. Such structures can be found in the vascular architecture (see Illustration 2b), for example, in which the glandular duct-like building principle works in conjunction with the plastic-synthetic principle. This is a section of kidney in which a knot of capillaries projects into the end of a glandular duct (Bowman's capsule).

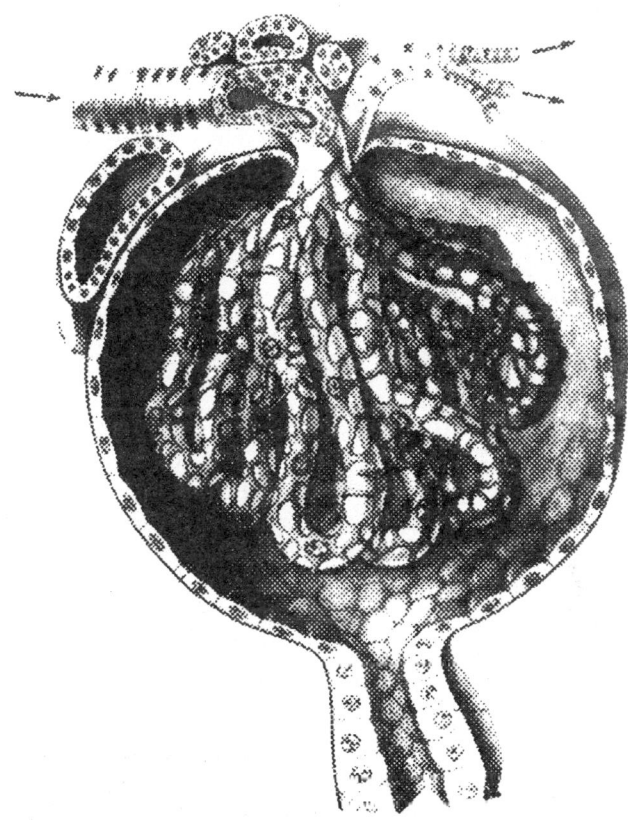

Illus. 2b: Kidney glomerulus with renal tubule as an example of the additive and plastic-synthetic principle. (Illus. 2 from: Bargmann, *Histologie und mikroskopische Anatomie des Menschen*, Thieme, Stuttgart 1962).

The cell reaches its last and greatest stage of deformation — and thereby the highest level in the architecture of the organism as a whole — in the nervous and sensory system. This decisive, highest step of deformation is characterized by the implantation of the previously extracellular fibrous structures into the cell itself. The higher structure does not arise outside the cell from expelled material, but within the cell itself. This leads to a further loss of vitality. These cells are no longer capable of division or regeneration, but there is an unbroken transition to those which have preserved greater vitality. In nerve cells the deformation has reached such a degree that a cell structure with a thickness of approximately 130° develops a thread-like, fibre-containing extension which can grow up to one metre in length. As far as length is concerned, such a cell belongs entirely in the macroscopic field. The only reason why it cannot be seen is because of its thickness. A similar development is also true of the lens fibres of the eye and the red blood corpuscles, in which the nucleus practically disappears. All these high-level deformations involve both the astral body and the 'I'. The latter not only brings about a reduction in the etheric life forces, but a greater withering and, in extreme cases, the death of the cells (see Illustration 3). This most extreme form of cell-deformation provides the basis for the highest level of histio-architecture that we know: the central nervous system. The principle involved in this structure is neither an additive one nor an extracellular plastic-synthetic one. On the contrary, this most complex stage of micro-architecture is achieved through a deformative transformation which directly affects the life and the form of the cell.

The gradual deformation of the cell allows us to see how the supersensory elements of the human being are active in the material which is absorbed as basic nourishment at conception. This material is then assimilated in a kind of 'digestive process', creating the material organism as shaped by the four elements of the human being. We can recognize an important principle which applies to human beings and also to the higher animals: the generative processes which we described as part of the cellular phase and which culminate in the complete human form, already contain elements of their own decline. We will

AIDS — THE DEADLY SEED

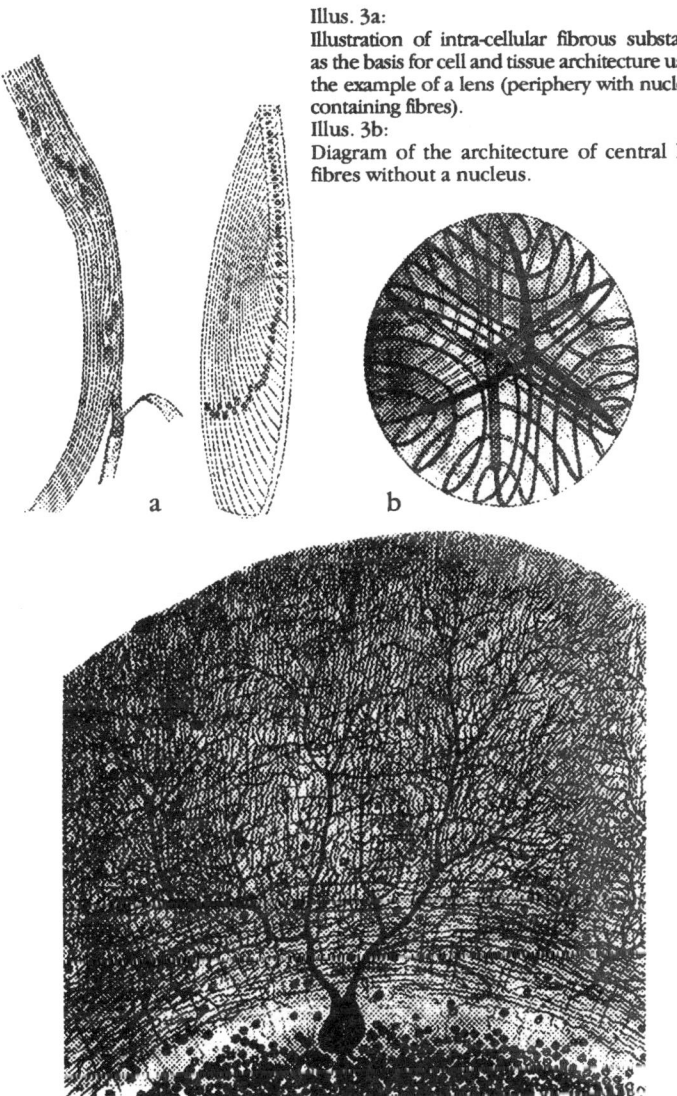

Illus. 3a:
Illustration of intra-cellular fibrous substance as the basis for cell and tissue architecture using the example of a lens (periphery with nucleus-containing fibres).

Illus. 3b:
Diagram of the architecture of central lens fibres without a nucleus.

Illus. 3c: Also-called Purkinje Cell in the cortex of the cerebellum as an example of radiating, fan-like cell architecture.

(Illus. 3a from: Rauber-Kopsch, *Lehrbuch und Atlas der Anatomie*, Vol. III, Thieme, Leipzig 1943. Illus. 3b and 3c from: Bargmann, *Histologie und mikroskopische Anatomie des Menschen*, Thieme, Stuttgart 1962).

encounter the same principle again in the humoural phase. Here the decline affects the individual existence of the cell, which progressively loses its vitality and original form at each new stage of disintegration for the benefit the human being it serves. The marks of the astral body and the 'I', which the cell carries only faintly on its surface at the lowest stage, penetrate the cell itself to an ever more fundamental degree at the later stages and deform it beyond recognition.

The construction of the human being through the metabolic stream — the external digestion

Let us now look at the humoural construction of the human being:

After birth human beings are open to three different processes from the environment, which enter into the three parts of the threefold organism [17]:

respiration	rhythmical system
nourishment	metabolic system
sensory impressions	nervous-sensory system

Let us start with nourishment, since at this stage we are interested in the aspect which builds up the organism.

We distinguish between external and internal nourishment. External nourishment has the aim — by oral, gastric and intestinal digestion — of putting organic matter, such as we find in plant and animal based foods, into the undifferentiated state which we have already encountered in the fertilization of the egg cell. This is the condition reached by the nutritional substance once everything resulting from the various elements which make up the plant and animal organism has been discarded. This state of formlessness is difficult to describe because it is only temporary, coming after the action of the higher elements but *preceding* the effects of external decay, fermentation,

---

[17] Rudolf Steiner, *The Case for Anthroposophy*, Rudolf Steiner Press, London 1970, Chapter Seven.

putrifaction, etc. Apart from preparation in the kitchen, the ego-organization is involved in breaking down the structure of our food through oral digestion. Here, food is distinguished both by smell and taste and subjected to the mechanical action of chewing. The astral body tends to dominate in the stomach (acidic phase) and the etheric body further down in the intestine (alkaline phase).

The liquid phase of the digestive process begins with insalivation and increases along the gastro-intestinal tract. A total of between four and six litres of liquid are injected and reabsorbed in the gastro-intestinal tract in 24 hours.[18]

Humoural circulation:
fluid organism-metabolism-protein

The *etheric body* acts on this fluid substance. It organizes the fluid in the organism as a whole, the percentage of which is reduced throughout life from more than 76% to somewhat more than 50%.[19] A middle-aged person weighing 75 kg will therefore consist of about 40 kg of water. The fluid in the body is active in the two areas which we described as cellular and humoural: 55% of fluid is tied to protein in the cell; the loss of this fluid, which occurs only rarely and with extreme dehydration, cannot be reversed; it is not compatible with life.[20] 45% of the fluid — bound to protein to a greater or lesser degree — circulates through the internal landscape of the organism, sluggishly or faster, steadily or rhythmically. It either seeps through the tissue or it flows in already formed ducts such as the lymphatic ducts, or it pulses rhythmically in the blood circulation. In the region of the head the flow of fluid shows a tendency to dam up, expanding into a lake, as it were, but always with a continuous inflow and outflow (brain and spinal fluid, eye chamber fluid).

There are active bursts of secretion from these circulating

---

18 Gauer/Kramer/Jung, *Physiologie des Menschen*, Vol. Eight, Chapter 'Ernährung, Verdauung, Intermediärstoffwechsel'. Munich/Berlin/Vienna 1970.
19 Ibid., Vol. Seven, Chapter 'Niere und Wasserhaushalt'.
20 Ibid.

internal fluids of the organism, in irregular phases determined by the intake of food. The secretions flow into the gastro-intestinal tract — as already explained — and return from there to the internal fluid circulation (enteral fluid circulation). The nourishment dissolved in them flows in and the etheric body uses the fluid circulation to carry what has been consumed to the inner organs, particularly to their constituent cells around which the fluid washes continuously. In this process a transition occurs from the spatially still measurable, extensive movement of the nutritional stream into a metabolic motion which can no longer be grasped in terms of space. What takes place, therefore, in the cells of the organism is outwardly in a state of rest but inwardly, i.e. biochemically, intensely active.[21]

The word 'metabolic' means the infinite number of continuing changes and transformations of substance which occur as movement; not extensively in space but in the 'intensive boundlessness'[22] which can only be described qualitatively: we have reached the centre of the etheric body in so far as it acts on matter in order to transform the undifferentiated substance of the external digestion into 'living substance'[23].

As well as the metabolic metamorphosis that takes place, a second characteristic of the etheric body can be identified here: namely the tendency for repetition, which we have already mentioned. It can be observed in the humoural circulation. The process always turns in on itself. But there is also an infinite amount of circular movement in such metabolic actions which are no longer spatially observable, where substances begin a process of transformation by which they eventually return to their starting point (biochemical metabolic cycles).

Finally, we may note that the etheric body and its function in fluid organization relies particularly on one substance which is capable of binding this fluid as living substance and which thereby becomes an elementary carrier of etheric life: protein.

21 J. Bockemühl (ed.), *Erscheinungsformen des Ätherischen, Beiträge zur Anthroposophie*, vol 1, Stuttgart 1985.
22 Rudolf Steiner, *Kunst und Kunsterkenntnis* (GA 271), Dornach 1961, lecture of 17 February 1918.
23 Rudolf Steiner and Ita Wegman, *Fundamentals of Therapy*, Chapter Five.

Breathing:
air organism–rhythm–the fats

In summary, the etheric construction of the human being unfolds in the alternation between two phases, the cellular and the humoural; that is to say, between 'stable and unstable protein'.[24]

This twofold process of building-up is now affected everywhere, although with different degrees of intensity, by the *astral body*. The astral body uses the air which enters the organism during respiration. In the same way that solid nutrients were introduced into the liquid phase 'from below' through oral, gastric and intestinal digestion, the gaseous ones enter the humoural stream of the blood 'from above'.

Just as the etheric body creates a continuous equilibrium in the fluids flowing through the tissues of the extra- and intracellular stock, so the astral body regulates the exchange of gases between the blood circulation and the tissues. The totality of all gases is ordered into the air organism just as the totality of organic liquids is organized into a fluid organism by the etheric body. And if the etheric body acts on the metabolic processes at the level of cells and tissues, the astral body acts on the rhythmical pulsations of the structures which it creates itself and which have been placed on a higher structural level through the deformative restructuring of the cell material. These are, above all, the structures comprising vessels, muscles and connective tissue in all their variations.

If the basic mode of the etheric body is a circular flowing movement, the basic mode of the astral body can be seen as the rhythmical alternation between internal and external. The etheric body finds its fulfilment in the flow of the internal fluids; the astral body must enter and leave the body by means of the respiratory process in order to maintain contact with the organic environment.

This polar span between inhalation and exhalation is vital to the astral body. It also clarifies how it acts on the regular and circulatory flow associated with the etheric body: namely through the pulse. The motion induced by the etheric body is sluggish;

24 Rudolf Steiner, *Geisteswissenschaftliche Gesichtspunkte zur Therapie* (GA 313), Dornach 1963, lecture of 16 April 1921.

indeed, it comes to rest — from a spatial point of view — at the centre of etheric action, i.e. at the boundary of the cell. The motion induced by the astral body increases in speed and in spatial extension the more the latter affects it. There is thus a clear polarity between the intensive motion at the centre of the metabolism and the spatially extensive motion of the musculature of the limbs. The pulsating circular movement of the blood mediates between the two.

The action of the astral body on the humoural substance raises the latter to a feeling level, it becomes 'feeling substance'.[25] Only substance which is grasped and transformed by the force which later forms consciousness, but prior to any processes of consciousness, can provide the basis for the development of consciousness. Just as protein belongs to the domain of the etheric body, so the fat metabolism belongs to the domain of the astral body.

Equilibrium:
warmth organism–homoeostasis–carbohydrates

The nutritional substance to build up our humoural system is made biologically available to human beings through the action of the ego-organization. Whereas water and air as elements of the etheric and astral bodies have to be extracted from the environment, warmth, as a medium of the 'I', is produced inside the organism.

This warmth, penetrated by the 'I', permeates the substance and it becomes 'spirit-supporting substance'.[26] The human organism has then achieved its full organization such that the intervention by the human 'I' through the will becomes possible. This requires the metabolic substance to be in a condition which permits the release of energy 'from above' — that is to say, through the will active in the soul. This intervention from above is only possible in a heat-producing organism which is organized by the ego.

[25] Rudolf Steiner and Ita Wegman, *Fundamentals of Therapy*, Chapter Five.
[26] Ibid.

Just as the etheric body works in the circulation, and the astral body in the rhythmical to and fro of breathing in the widest sense, the 'I' works in the production of organic *homoeostasis*. What does this mean?

Nourishment, movement, respiration and sense impressions all cause continuous change in the equilibrium of the internal systems. The restoration of this equilibrium throughout the system — in the intestines, blood, tissue and organs — is due to the ego-organization. Thus it regulates the presence of substances and their functional effects in the blood and other areas of the organism. The build up and metabolism of the carbohydrates are directly under its control.

Stages of decomposition —
releasing the soul element from the body

The construction of the organism from a humoural point of view, as we have described it above, is now supplemented by a process of decomposition analogous to that which takes place in the cellular phase. There, too, a process of decomposition caused by the astral body, and to an even greater extent by the 'I', is built into the cell architecture — which is initially constructed mainly by the etheric body — and this can be recognized by the gradual deformation of the cell. Similarly, a process of decomposition is active in the humoural phase. It affects substance which has been transformed into energy and causes what has been built up to leave the body through the reverse process which starts at this point.

The initially self-contained organism, which is so impressive in human beings and animals, transcends itself through the metabolic changes leading to decomposition. The structures which have been altered by decomposition in the cellular phase remain in the organism for the duration of its life. They form the permanent stock of the human body. By contrast, the substances which are continuously fed into the body as nutrition during the humoural phase, leave the body again by means of 'excretion' — using the term in the widest sense. During decomposition the organism excretes not only substances, but also liberates the *soul and spiritual components* which are present in the organism on an unconscious level through the action of its supersensory elements. The organism transcends its organic boundaries and enters the sphere of *consciousness*. The related phenomena can be classified as follows:

The *will* as a function of the soul is liberated by the action of the 'I' in organic *combustion*. The creation of physical heat and the will in the soul are different components of the same process of decomposition. The carbohydrates are central to these combustion processes connected with the will.

Feeling as a second soul function is released through the degenerative action of the astral body in the *respiratory* processes of the organism. After all, the carbon dioxide exhaled by the astral body through the lungs is only an expression of the matter burned by the 'I'. In this sense the burning and respiratory functions of the 'I' and the astral body are very closely linked. We can also say that the 'I', by burning carbohydrates, assists the astral body by enabling it to exhale carbon dioxide. Carbon dioxide is created essentially through the combustion of carbohydrates, and this combustion in turn has an external effect by serving the energy needs of the muscles. The astral body for its part assists the 'I' by offering it the fats it has built up for combustion, which enables the 'I' to maintain the steady body temperature of the organism.

But a trace of decomposition can be found even in the etheric body, which otherwise appears to act only constructively. We might describe it as a *withering*. It tends to be found in the cellular phase rather than in the humoural one. A definite withering can be found on a cellular level in the nervous system in particular, when it loses vitality. But loss of vitality means the liberation of ether, which does not, however, disappear but is made available by the etheric body to the astral body and the 'I' for the soul function of *imagination*. A corresponding degenerative process in the humoural area affected by the etheric body can be understood as follows: the etheric body would not of its own accord release the liquid it has taken in but would preserve it in the internal circulation which it regulates. Here the action of the astral body (together with the 'I') forces the fluid out through perspiration and urination.

Finally, we find a specific form of decomposition in situations where the *physical* structures become almost devoid of life, in other words, where they practically die. This is the case with the sensory organs. These structures, which have been integrated into the physical body through the degenerative action of the external world, in turn liberate the mental action of *observation* in the consciousness.

The following representation (Diagram 3) is a summary of the relationships described above.

Diagram 3

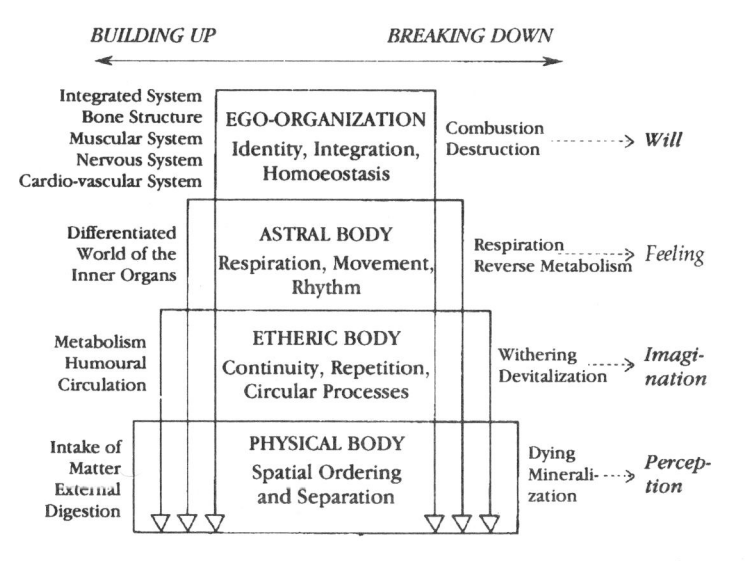

BUILDING UP ←		BREAKING DOWN →	
Integrated System Bone Structure Muscular System Nervous System Cardio-vascular System	**EGO-ORGANIZATION** Identity, Integration, Homoeostasis	Combustion Destruction ·······>	*Will*
Differentiated World of the Inner Organs	**ASTRAL BODY** Respiration, Movement, Rhythm	Respiration ·······> Reverse Metabolism	*Feeling*
Metabolism Humoural Circulation	**ETHERIC BODY** Continuity, Repetition, Circular Processes	Withering ·······> Devitalization	*Imagi- nation*
Intake of Matter External Digestion	**PHYSICAL BODY** Spatial Ordering and Separation	Dying Minerali- ·······> zation	*Percep- tion*

Natural science–spiritual science.
Complementary knowledge

Looking back at the epistemological situation of the natural sciences (see Chapter One) we can ask the following question: Is complementary knowledge possible? Does it rest on a methodologically sound base? Can the distortion of reality introduced into our view of the world by object-bound thinking be rectified by supersensory knowledge?

It could be, after all, that crossing the boundary of objective consciousness into the supersensory world initially takes us in a completely different direction from the world disclosed by instrumental observation in the biological-anthropological field.

'When we study ordinary science we start either with the simplest living organisms or with the simplest life form, the cell. Then we progress from the simple stage to more complex ones, that is to say, we ascend from the stages nearest to simple, purely physical matter to the highly complex human organism. But when we pursue the science of the spirit at a serious level we start from the other end, as it were; we descend from study of the spiritual aspect of the cosmos and regard this spiritual aspect as the complex element. We regard the cell as the simplest element in the organism. From the perspective of the science of the spirit, the cosmos is exceedingly complex. And in the same way that we add to the complexity of our knowledge as we proceed from the cell to the human being, we simplify the knowledge we gain in the cosmos until we come to the human being. We follow opposite paths, i.e. we proceed from opposite starting points. But by pursuing the science of the spirit in this way, we do not touch on the areas which comprise the sensory empiricism of today. It is of great importance that there should be no misunderstanding in these matters of principle. That is why I have to ask you to excuse me if I sound pedantic to you today. It would be a great mistake for someone to think: well, it is rather useless to conduct empirical studies in physiology and biology; why do we need specialist sciences; people simply need to develop spiritual capabilities, to look into the spiritual world in order to understand how human beings function — how sick and healthy human beings function — and then to establish a spiritual science of medicine. Some people take such an attitude today but it leads nowhere. The only result is that they complain mightily about empirical medicine, but they are complaining about something of which they have no knowledge. It is not a question of drawing a line at ordinary, sensory, empirical science and founding a science of the spirit which comes from spiritual cloud-cuckoo-land. That is not how things are in relation to the empirical sciences, i.e. what are called the empirical sciences today, but what I would like to call here the sensory, empirical sciences. It is not like that at all. For example, when you undertake research in the science of the spirit you will not make the same discoveries as research undertaken with the microscope. You would be quite justified in considering someone a charlatan if he tried to make you believe that he could discover the same things in the science of the spirit as can be discovered with the microscope. That is not so. The results of empirical research as it is understood today are valid. We must not discard the sensory empirical elements if we want to make science more complete in the sense of the science of the spirit, of Anthroposophy, but we must take them into account. Someone who is a specialist — if I may use this word — in anthroposophical spiritual science will not find anything to make him think that there is not an even greater necessity to undertake the sensory, empirical study of the phenomena in the world in his pursuit of Anthroposophy.' [27]

Earlier we described observation and thinking as the 'two arms of consciousness'. Our arms can reach in both directions. But just as the arms extend from a *single* organism, they can be brought together from opposite directions and linked. Linking arms gives the person who does so an enhanced feeling of the reality of the 'I' in his body — a basic intuition of self. Arms of consciousness which reach into the world are able to achieve an intuitive understanding of the realities of the world when they are linked, an intuitive understanding which is brought about by complementary knowledge. This intuitive understanding of reality can never be assured in advance, that is to say, through theoretical considerations; it can only be experienced in research on a case by case, step by step basis through direct evidence. With the particular phenomenon discussed here — the nature of the human being — this cognitive process leads us to conclude that subsensory observation using instruments to investigate ever smaller phenomena can be made

[27] Rudolf Steiner, *Physiologisch — Therapeutisches auf Grundlage der Geisteswissenschaft* (GA 314), Dornach 1975, lecture of 26 October 1922. Available in English as *Fundamentals of Anthroposophical Medicine*, Mercury Press, Spring Valley, New York 1986.

complete by supersensory knowledge of the human being's constituent elements. The contexts which are reduced and increasingly cast aside in the process of instrumental observation are rediscovered when the boundary to supersensible knowledge is crossed. We can thus complete the diagram from the first chapter in a complementary sense (see Diagram 4):

Diagram 4

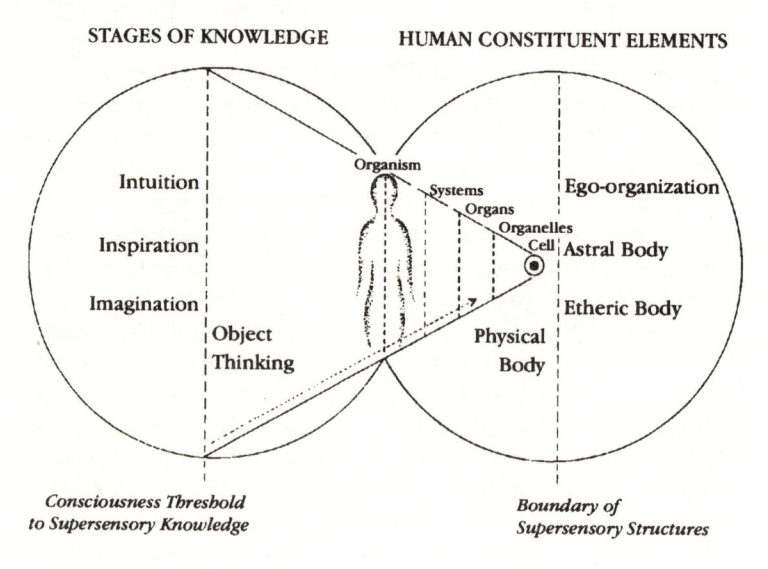

STAGES OF KNOWLEDGE   HUMAN CONSTITUENT ELEMENTS

- Intuition
- Inspiration
- Imagination
- Object Thinking

Organism, Systems, Organs, Organelles, Cell

- Ego-organization
- Astral Body
- Etheric Body
- Physical Body

Consciousness Threshold to Supersensory Knowledge

Boundary of Supersensory Structures

CHAPTER THREE

THE BIOLOGICAL INDIVIDUAL

In the extended concept of medicine as understood through Anthroposophy, the multitude of human illnesses is ordered by a conceptual framework for understanding their symptoms. Numerous hypotheses about the nature of the human being are available to this end. They are the result of anthroposophical research and can be used in medical practise as the conceptual apparatus for an understanding of pathological processes. As a consequence, the anthroposophical framework of ideas and the wealth of natural scientific knowledge supplement one another through 'complementary knowledge'.[28] This leads to a completely new expansion and deepening of medical science which goes beyond the findings of the natural sciences.

The *fourfold* constitution of the human being and the threefold nature of the organism are particularly significant within the wealth of conceptual models provided by an anthroposophical anthropology. We have already discussed the fourfold division from a medical perspective in Chapter Two. At this point let us look at the threefold structure of the organism so that we can subsequently throw some light on the nature of the immunological processes.

The threefold structure of the human organism — a key concept

The idea of the threefold structure of the organism helps us to understand the fundamental pathological processes in human beings. If this idea is linked with the four constituent elements from which the human being is constructed, we have the most

---

28 See Chapter One.

important tools used by anthroposophical medicine. This basic anthropological idea, which was developed by Rudolf Steiner, has the same scientific significance as the idea of the archetypal plant had for Goethe in understanding the nature of plants.[29] The idea of the threefold structure is just as invisible 'to the eye'[30] as that of the archetypal plant. It has to be conceived as an idea. But then it can be re-cognized through observation in the innumerable permutations of its morphological and functional manifestations in any examination of the human organism. It can be demonstrated in the organism, as it were. Even the terms used to describe the three morphological and functional constituents:

    nervous and sensory system
    rhythmical cardio-pulmonary system
    metabolic and limb system

are taken from the areas in which the conceptual constituents are essentially manifest.

A first, elementary 'reading' of this idea of the threefold structure is provided by the human skeleton. The basic form of the skeleton shows the organism to be constructed out of the polarity of the enclosed cavity of the head and the radiating limbs. The skeletal structure of the thorax (thoracic cavity) mediates between the two with both a rounded, enclosing and a radiating, extending principle of construction at work.[31]

If we move beyond the skeletal arrangement and include the total morphological and functional structure, we find the following: the three components of the organism appear as three body cavities built one above the other: the abdominal, thoracic and head cavities. The structures of head and thoracic cavities are, from an anatomical viewpoint, clearly separated from one another; the thoracic and abdominal cavities less so. The latter two are separated without the direct involvement of the skeleton. These cavities create internal space. The internal body cavities and the external environment enter into a unique relationship with one another in each of the three components:

29 Rudolf Steiner, *The Case for Anthroposophy*, Chapter Seven.
30 J.W. von Goethe, "Glückliches Ereignis", in: *Naturwissenschaftliche Schriften*, vol.1, ed. Rudolf Steiner.
31 Rudolf Steiner, *The Study of Man*, Rudolf Steiner Press, London 1975, lecture 10.

Diagram 5

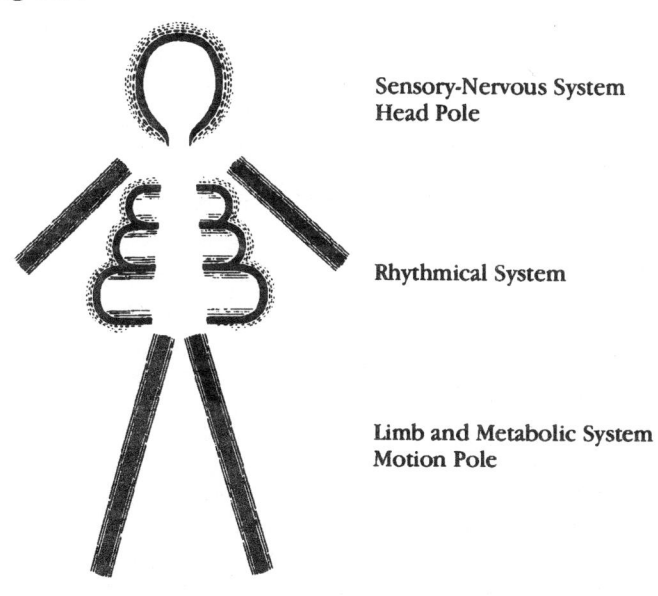

Sensory-Nervous System
Head Pole

Rhythmical System

Limb and Metabolic System
Motion Pole

The head cavity is the centre of the *nervous and sensory system*. Here the orientation of the relationship with the environment is from the outside to the inside, essentially passive receptivity. We give this function the general term *perception*. Like 'gulfs' (Rudolf Steiner) the external world, foreign to the inner organism, reaches into the individual world of the head and penetrates further inward along the nerves. The sensory organs and the central nervous system are thus components of an integrated network of organs. The culmination of the central nervous system in the inner organ of the brain and the sensory organs with their orientation from outside to inside are pointing in the same direction; they are functionally concordant.

This is not the case with the abdominal cavity and the associated limbs. Here we find the centre of the *metabolic and limb system*. The opposite direction predominates: the limbs reach into the external world from the internal base of the organism. Their general function is *movement*. The internal space in which the inward facing 'intensive infinity' (Rudolf Steiner) of the metabolic motion takes place, and the limbs which are externally active in extensive motion represent a functional polarity — although they are related in the same way as the senses and nerves. They are morphologically and functionally discordant.

The polarity of the head cavity (passive receptivity) and the limbs (active grasping) therefore contains two further polarities (the senses and nerves and the metabolism and limbs). Here there is an apparent imbalance — at least when we consider the outward shape: the enclosed internal space of the head dominates above while the outward-reaching activity of the limbs dominates below.

The *rhythmical system,* which mediates between these two poles, is apparent in both the respiratory system and in cardiac activity as the steady, rhythmically ordered alternation of motion from outside to inside and inside to outside.

If we look at the specific actions of the organism at the poles of the nervous and sensory system and the metabolic and limb system we can observe the following: in the *metabolic system* the 'I' and the other human constituent elements act on substance in a way which makes it into an integral part of the organism. We dealt with the stages of this humoural process in Chapter Two. We saw how the external digestion liberates nutrients from the forms imposed by extra-human biological entities in nature. They have to pass through a stage which we identified as 'undifferentiated'. Therefore, at the boundary between external and internal digestion, the foreign *form* is rejected but the *substance* is accepted. Digestion can be described as this dual function of *rejection of form* and acceptance of *substance.* The 'I', then, works in opposite directions in the digestive process. It breaks down and destroys the external, formed nutrients, but it builds up and shapes the undifferentiated nutritional substance. The ingestion of the stream of humoural substance by the biological individual and its component elements thus leads to the *self-representation of the biological 'I'* in the undifferentiated substance. The latter is gradually overcome and 'incorporated' completely in the metabolic process. This overcoming and complete domination of substance through the formative forces of the biological self is one of the fundamental prerequisites for organic health in the metabolic sphere. This is the human 'life pole'. The 'lower' human organs — that is, the organs of the metabolic system which extends throughout the body from its centre in the abdominal cavity — wholly serve the purpose of the biological individual's self-representation in substance. In this sense the metabolic system can also be described as the 'substance pole' of the human being.

The *limb system* is engaged in comparable, but external, activity. Here, too, matter is deprived of its natural form — in the manufacturing process, for example — and transformed into something quite different after passing through an undifferentiated stage: a workpiece, a product or a work of art. The dual phases of this kind of productive work by the limbs correspond directly with the dual phases of external and internal digestion.

Given the fundamental affinity between these processes, the polarity which exists between metabolism and limbs lies primarily in the purpose and nature of their motion. In the metabolic system, the chemical transformations (motions) lead to repetitive, circular biochemical processes — 'intensive infinity'. In contrast, the arbitrary and impulsive extensive motion of the limbs is fragmentary in nature. The limbs tend to disrupt the completeness of the environment. Only occasionally do they develop a self-contained whole out of the fragments created by their destruction of the world.

In the *nervous system,* we do not take in and assimilate substance, but form, structure. Here the sensory organs and the nervous system work concordantly so that the *substance* of the external world is rejected and only the outside *form* is assimilated. It is possible to demonstrate how every sensory organ fulfils this dual function. The inflow of sensory impressions can be seen to be a flow of *in-formation.* [32] Just as the nutritional stream in the metabolism is tied to the humoural phase of the organism, so is the flow of sensory information tied to the cellular phase. This flow of information is free of matter; it penetrates the sensory and nervous system as changes of state on the surface of an infinitely interlinked cellular network (of neurons). And as the organism is built up 'from below' via the humoural stream, the breakdown of the organism takes place in the formative impulse 'from above' through the network of the sensory and nervous system.

32 Johannes Rohan, *Funktionelle Anatomie des Menschen,* Stuttgart 1984.

The body is 'open' from below through nutrition; continuous humoural build-up is introduced from below into the system of circulating fluids. But it is also 'open' from above, because the cellular breakdown which originates in the cephalic system draws into it — above all in the waking state — the informational and sensory flow arising from perception. Consciousness is built up on the basis of this breakdown. The awakening consciousness is filled with forms which enter from outside through the senses. The biological self-representation of the 'I' in the metabolism is therefore supplemented by the *representation of the world in consciousness*.

It is of some relevance to compare the construction of world representation in consciousness with the building up of self-representation in the organism. We described the process of nourishment in two phases. The shape and the formal traces of foreign substance are rejected in the external digestion. The substance itself enters an undifferentiated stage. Beyond this threshold it serves to build up the biological self (internal digestion). In sensory perception, the formal elements are separated from the entities or objects of the sensory world. The invasion of consciousness by the environment through perception forces the mental self to subjugate itself to the forms imposed by what is taken in; the 'evidence of the senses' cannot be denied. As consciousness is built up in further stages, the conscious 'I' is increasingly free to make use of these perceptual elements. The 'I', liberated from its organic constraints through the disintegration occurring in the sensory and nervous system, can 'combine' perceptual elements at will. But consciousness reaches its highest level when these self-conscious thought processes actively submit to the non-physical forms of cosmic thought. If this submission is complete, the 'I' can realize itself completely in the forms of the world. We call the result of the total submission of the self to the representation of the world through thinking, *the truth*. The construction of consciousness therefore includes a passage through three stages: the representation of the world through the senses (perception), free combination of percepts, and finally, representation of the world in the thinking process (concepts).

While the total submission of substance to the self-representation of the 'I' in the unconscious metabolism always occurs naturally under normal conditions, the equivalent process in the higher human being is a matter of freedom. Truth is not a natural state but a moral aim which can be pursued in freedom. But the organs of the nervous system, located in the head cavity and spreading from there to the rest of the body, serve to represent the forms of the outside world in the interior of the organism. In this respect the nervous and sensory system is the 'formal pole' in human beings.

The processes of the 'I' and its constituent elements in the metabolism are unconscious because it is deeply immersed in matter. Mental and metabolic activity are identical in this process and cannot be separated. Human beings are asleep as far as self-representation in the body is concerned. By contrast, the constituent elements of the human being surmount their organic constraints through the disintegration which occurs in the nervous and sensory system. At this formal pole there is a clear distinction between conscious mental activity and the imprint of this activity in the nervous and sensory organs.

We have already seen how the structures of the nervous and sensory system are moulded by the human constituent elements down to a cellular level and that external sensory impressions are involved in this process. Sensory experience contributes to the formation of the brain.[33] This process was described as the climax of the processes of organic breakdown. The head is therefore not only the formal pole but also the 'death pole' in human beings.[34] Nevertheless, organic disintegration has the simultaneous effect of releasing the human constituent elements, and as a consequence they can join in the free action of the processes of consciousness.

Through its independent intermediary position, the *rhythmical system* imparts a dreamlike consciousness. On the one hand, the latter is filled with the self-experience of the body, yet perceptual images of the world are haphazardly mixed in with it. The relationship between the human constituent elements and their

---

33 Rudolf Steiner, *The Education of the Child*, Rudolf Steiner Press, London 1975.
34 Cf. Brothers Grimm: *The Godfather Death*.

material organization can be characterized in this 'intermediary system' by the steady rhythmical alternation of connection and disconnection, immersion and separation.

Specific capacities of the soul are linked with these various levels of consciousness in the organism's three elements: the will and the instincts arise in the metabolic system and exist in an almost sleeplike state of consciousness. Feelings, with their particular characteristics, arise from the rhythmical immersion and separation of the human constituent elements in the middle human being. Waking ideas and, above all, perceptions transcend the rigidifying forms of degeneration in the nervous and sensory system and thus lead an independent life in the consciousness (see Diagram 6).

In summary, this short sketch of the threefold division of the organism shows that every biological form, every organic structure in the human being, participates in the nervous and sensory system if the latter is understood not merely as a system of specific organs but as the form-giving pole within the context of the threefold structure. By contrast, every motion, every metabolic change is fundamentally invisible, formless, a pure process. The metabolic and limb system is present wherever motion and change occur in the organism if, once again, we conceive of it as the conceptual antithesis of the form-giving pole. A system must mediate between these two poles to provide a balance. *Rhythm* is the term we use for the regularly structured compensation between two opposing motions. The idea of rhythm is apparent throughout the organism. Rhythm acts to prevent the two poles described above from falling apart, but it also prevents their confrontation without any mediating influence. The organism would fall ill without such rhythm. The rhythmical system is the built-in 'healer' of these polar pathological tendencies. [35]

It becomes clear that the nervous system, the rhythmical system and the metabolic and limb system must be understood as functional categories within the threefold structure, and not as parts of the anatomy. It is a *conceptual structure* which penetrates and is effective throughout the organism. In other words: the organism is divided into three, not physically but *conceptually*. Rudolf Steiner

---

35 Rudolf Steiner, *Man as Symphony of the Creative Word*, Rudolf Steiner Press, London 1970, lecture 10.

AIDS — THE DEADLY SEED

Diagram 6

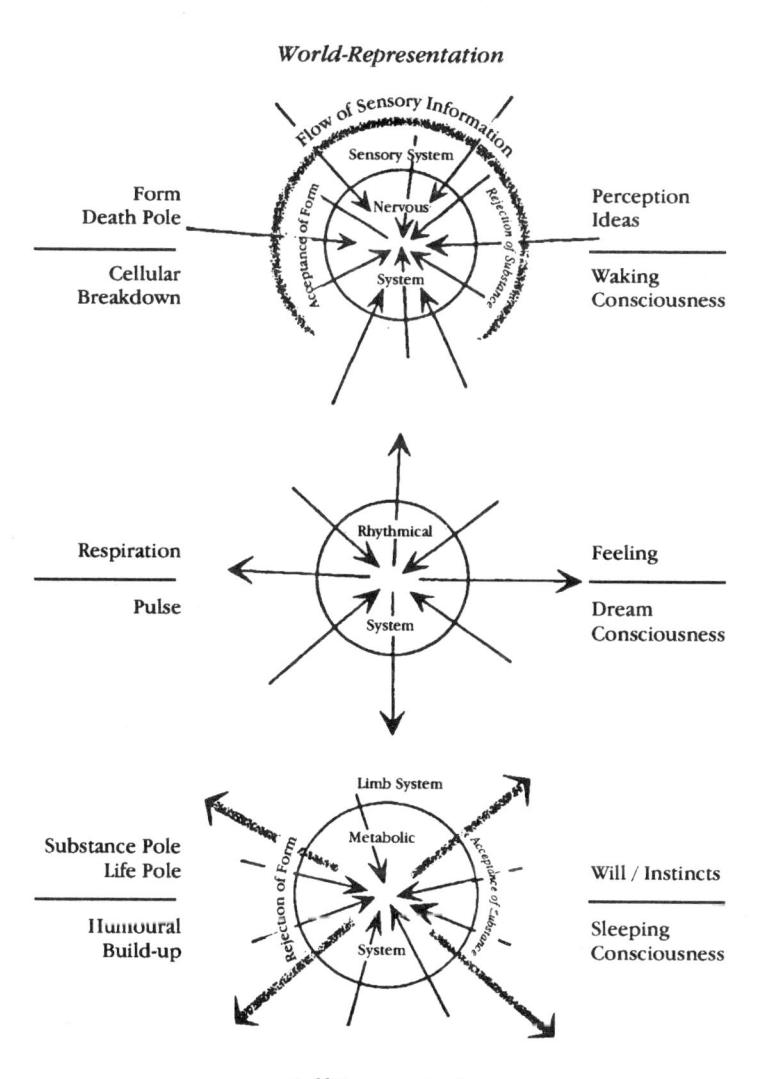

World-Representation

Form Death Pole	Perception Ideas
Cellular Breakdown	Waking Consciousness

(Sensory System / Nervous System — Flow of Sensory Information, Acceptance of Form, Rejection of Substance)

Respiration	Feeling
Pulse	Dream Consciousness

(Rhythmical System)

Substance Pole Life Pole	Will / Instincts
Humoural Build-up	Sleeping Consciousness

(Limb System / Metabolic System — Rejection of Form, Acceptance of Substance)

Self-Representation

once said the following in this sense: 'People think of the head as being there at the top, and they assume that when a man is decapitated he has no head left. It is not so, however; a man is substantially [i.e. as sensory perception, *K.D.*] head all over. Even right to the end of his big toe he is head, for his head sends down its substance there. ... If through vigorous auto-suggestion of a negative kind we can suggest away the head of a man, so that in appearance he is headless, and if we can do this not only in thought but so that we really see the man as headless, then the rest of his organism also disappears; with the head goes the whole of the man as being perceptible to the senses.' [36]

The biological individual

Every living organism represents a 'biological individual', in the first instance in the commonplace sense that the daisy which grows 'here' is different from the one which grows 'there'. They are two different specimens of the same species. The species, i.e. the reason why we recognize and describe all the different specimens as daisies, can only be grasped by conceptualization. It is common to all specimens. The specimen, however, has to be grasped by observation of the 'here' and 'there'. The concept of the species identifies the form, specific behaviour or function of the species; observation of the specimen is delineated by the boundaries of place and time within which the specimen materially appears. While an individual species appears in the multiplicity of its specimens as the unifying factor common to all, the single specimen is in the strictest sense 'unique'.

All specimens of a species should therefore be completely similar. But that is not the case. Although the formal and functional consistency of the specimens originates with the single species which determines them all, they nevertheless vary in time and space. All specimens of a species display a variety (variance) within a population as well as changes wrought by biological descent (generations). Variance can therefore be observed both spatially

---

[36] Rudolf Steiner, *The Evolution of Consciousness*, Rudolf Steiner Press, London 1979, lecture 5.

and consecutively in time. There can be two causes of variance. If the cause of variance lies in the numerous environmental influences, either natural or artificial, which affect every single specimen, only the individual specimen is ever affected. We can see how it has changed when compared with a neighbouring specimen within a population. Thus the features of a species (phenotype) vary from specimen to specimen. This environmentally determined variation in the phenotype contrasts with the underlying constancy of the species. The appearance of the individual daisy may vary, it may be flowering 'here', blossoming 'there' and wilting somewhere else; its appearance may vary in good or bad soil, in a valley or on a hill. The species, on the basis of which we recognize it as a daisy, remains constant. But there is one outside influence which penetrates deeper than appearance, than the phenotype, and that is fertilization. Fertilization not only changes the individual fertilized specimen, but all further specimens which are derived from it. This specific intervention — in contrast to arbitrary and unspecific environmental influences — brings about variance of a different kind. We can call it the genetic variance of a plant or an animal. In contrast to environmentally determined variance, which is restricted to the individual specimen, genetic variance is spread over the temporal progression of generations of specimens. We call the rules which govern this influence — heredity. Genetic variance is not always caused by fertilization. There are also spontaneous changes in the nature of a species which are then inherited, so-called mutations. In this respect three different causes of variance have been identified: environmental influences on the phenotype, sexual fertilization and mutation.

Just as with environmentally determined variance, genetic variance can be brought about through artificial intervention, as well as occurring by natural means. The former ranges from directed breeding or cultivation via genetic engineering to mutation by means of radiation. Artificial mutation always results in a deformation of the phenotype.

If the species takes on a specific appearance, as it were, with each specimen, it demonstrates in the succession of the generations the spread of its genetic variation within the area of constancy of the genotype. Where the individual specimen only displays the phenotype, the generational pattern shows the genotype of a species. The individual phenotypic specimen is spatially restricted to the 'here' or 'there' — as we saw. Equally, it has temporal restrictions: in annual or perennial plants, for example, through cotyledon and fruit; with the higher animals through conception and death. By contrast, the individual nature of the species is present in successive generations as the genotype. Once it dies, each unique specimen has gone. But the species continues by maintaining the constancy of its specific nature (germ line).

If we look at specimens from the perspective of the species, they appear to be the dead ends of development in relation to the continuity of the species, to which the latter returns again at the death of each of its specimens. The individual specimen detaches itself from the germ line of the species and develops its individually unique nature in space and time, its biological 'destiny'.

The individual nature of the species, which has to be conceptualized, and the uniqueness of the specimen, which only becomes evident to sensory observation in time and space, interpenetrate in each single organism encountered. We can call the result of this interpenetration the *biological individual*.

Since there is considerable variation in the degree to which the characteristic form of each species imposes itself on the matter which constitutes the specimen, the rank of the biological individual also varies. This becomes evident in the hierarchy of the organisms, among both plants and animals. The biological individual expresses itself only weakly in the lower organisms, but increasingly more strongly in the higher ones. This is evident in the fact that with each higher stage of development the individual specimen becomes increasingly more significant in relation to the species as a whole. A greater degree of individuality in a specimen is an expression and measure of higher development in plants and animals.

The biological individual is developed most strongly in human beings because the relationship between species and specimen reaches a new level. [37] While plant and animal species subsume a wealth of specimens, the individual specimen subsumes the

---

37   Cf. Rudolf Bubner, *Evolution, Reinkarnation, Christentum*, Stuttgart 1975, and *Christologie und Evolution*, Stuttgart 1985.

species in human beings. The relationship is reversed. For each person is a species *sui generis* in respect of the spirit and appears as a unique specimen. He is 'incarnated'.[38] When the species becomes the specimen — as in human beings — the biological individual also reaches its highest form.

Sexual reproduction — an artifice of nature

The causes of environmentally determined variance in single specimens are generally clear. But how does the species produce the wealth of its genetic variance? How does it demonstrate the range of its possibilities within populations and generations? It uses the artifice of sexual reproduction. Sexual reproduction separates the daughter specimen from the mother specimen through a profound division and each time sets a new beginning which enables original intervention by the species in the unbroken continuity of the germ line. If we knew only *one* specimen of a species, the range of its variance would remain hidden from us. But if we get to know many specimens we learn more and more about the range of variance of the species concerned. Sexual reproduction enables the species gradually to measure out the area of its variance and to make visible the range of its possibilities. It is decisive in this respect that this artifice of nature, which appears in organisms as sexual fertilization, allows the biological individual to emerge more strongly than in asexual reproduction.

Thus sexual reproduction is inserted between the uniqueness of the specimen and the constant characteristics of the species as an artifice intended to bring out the range in variance of the latter.

Biological self and non-self

The process of higher development apparent in the inner process of differentiation in the construction and function of organisms, which is made possible by the artifice of sexual reproduction, requires that the individual structure separates itself from and

---

38 Cf. Rudolf Steiner, *Theosophy*, Chapter Two.

becomes independent of its external environment much more distinctly. The 'self' of an organism defines itself ever more sharply in the course of its higher development from the 'non-self' of its natural environment, but also from other organisms of the same species. Organs from a foreign biological self which is nevertheless of the same species are therefore perceived as 'alien' when they are transferred into the recipient organism — so-called organ transplantation — and are rejected.

But such separation of self and non-self cannot and must not lead to the total isolation of the organism from its environment. On the contrary, there is a great deal of interaction between the biological individual and its environment. To maintain this paradox of strict autonomy on the one hand and constant exchange between biological organisms and their environment on the other calls for extraordinary artifices of nature. The whole subject of immunology in modern medicine is concerned with these 'artifices'. [39] It is therefore understandable if some scientists almost equate the secret of life with that of immunology. The secret of life is indeed expressed in this paradox. The way in which immunological processes have determined the shape of modern knowledge, which is still engaged in continuous change and expansion, is — like all modern biology and medicine — unthinkable without the immense experimental expansion and strengthening of the observational element at a cellular and subcellular level. Let us pursue this advance of observation into the unknown in the direction of the immunological processes.

Immunology — a biological learning process

In the eighteenth century, it was discovered in Scotland that farmers who through constant contact with their cattle were contracting cowpox, which is harmless in humans, were noticeably often spared from smallpox. They were immune. This experience was put to use in smallpox vaccination. It was discovered only later that throughout life natural immunity is built up to a whole range of foreign organisms, which was

[39] R. Keller, *Immunologie und Immunpathologie*, Stuttgart 1981.

described as 'occult immunization'. What had happened?

Having to deal with the germs of disease leaves the organism in an altered state. After renewed contact with the same germs, the reaction which occurred the first time does not recur. The initial sensitivity has been lifted. The organism has acquired immunity as a result of the first contact.

This purely biological process, which takes place at an unconscious level ('occult'), can be compared to processes in consciousness. When a person is stimulated by something which was unknown to him before, the process begins which we call *learning*. The learning process changes the way a person is in relation to his state *before* the single or repeated perception. There are many different forms and stages to this change, which takes place in somewhat different ways in children and adults. Broadly speaking, three such stages can be described:

— *Memory development:* An experience is retained in a manner which allows it to be reproduced for external or internal reasons. A person has an initial experience and is altered by it to the extent that when the stimulus is repeated, the old experience can be recalled to memory. Thus an immense stock of experiences accumulates throughout life which forms the substratum for voluntary or involuntary memory acts.

— This elementary stage of learning precedes a more advanced capacity of consciousness, which is *the ability to form judgements*. At this stage experience is not only preserved but inwardly assimilated, integrated to become part of the personality as a whole. Memory growth itself does not initiate a change of personality but the method of assimilating experiences which we call *judgement* does. The more judgements we have formed in coming to terms with the world, the more comprehensive is the soul with its individual accumulation of world experience.

— The last stage in coming to terms with the world through the learning process is *skill*. The acquisition of skills represents the innermost transformation of experience. The human 'I' can do something which it could not do before, not only because it has developed memory and formed judgements in its contact with the world, but because it has acquired a new skill. Thus the process of learning as a whole passes over into action through the eye of the needle of the self.

The relationship between mental and biological learning

Such a learning process also takes place on an organic and unconscious level between the biological 'I' and the non-'I' of the environment. The organism constantly encounters animate and inanimate foreign matter, not only when it may carry smallpox, measles or other infectious diseases. At the same time processes of organic memory formation, formation of judgement and skill acquisition occur. That is why we speak of immunological memory, immunological recognition (judgement) and immunological resistance (skill). In contact with the environment the organism not only 'learns' to distinguish 'I' from non-'I', but also to remember specific encounters with foreign material and in equally specific defensive reactions to mobilize its own organic self and hold its ground against foreign material. At first glance the comparison between the conscious learning stages which we sketched out and the stages of immunological interaction between biological self and non-self appears to rest on a vague analogy which has only hermeneutical relevance. But complementary knowledge sees both processes embedded in the activity of the same supersensory human constituent elements. They become comparable because of their common basic structure arising from these elements. Thus individual learning stages can be assigned to the various constituent elements in accordance with the latter's characteristics.

— *Perception* is a function of the 'I' at the physical level.
— *Memory*, in contrast, is tied to the time-body (etheric body).[40]

[40] Rudolf Steiner, *At the Gates of Spiritual Science*, Rudolf Steiner Press, London 1970, lecture 14.

— *Judgement,* in which a specifically orientated meeting between person and world takes place, belongs to the astral body. For the latter forms judgements from its alternating submersion into the self and the outside world. [41]

In biological learning, the human constituent elements are immersed in the organic matter; they give it the function and morphological structure which the study of biology reveals. In the case of learning as an intellectual process, our attention is directed to a greater degree toward the activity of the human constituent elements which have freed themselves from their organic ties. We saw this liberation of the constituent elements in connection with the processes of organic disintegration (see Chapter Two).

To sum up, the biological individual, the organic self and its immunity, can be seen as follows: the artifice of combining full 'openness' and strict autonomy presupposes something which we have already encountered in describing the human threefold structure. We need to consider this again:

Digestion decomposes foreign biological matter insofar as it serves as nourishment. The form, which originates with the type of plant or animal nourishment, is rejected during digestion and only the undifferentiated substance is absorbed. Whenever this decomposition is unsuccessful or incomplete, *poisoning* takes place. Digestion is thus also detoxification. In this respect a foreign organism which penetrates the biological self without this decomposition taking place acts as a poison.

However, foreign biological organisms can enter the organism parenterally (by-passing the digestive tract); they do not serve as nourishment and are therefore not digested as they should be. They include, above all, micro-organisms. A different kind of decomposition of which the organism is capable comes into play in the process by which the biological self deals with these foreign biological entities: *recognition.* In organic recognition the structure is perceived and the substance is rejected — the reverse of digestion. If this decomposition is not completely

---

[41] Rudolf Steiner, *Von Seelenrätseln* (GA 21), Dornach 1976, Chapter Three and Chapter Four/Five.

successful a different kind of poisoning takes place which we call *infection*. Immunity, then, is the detoxifying ability of the organism through recognition and rejection of a foreign entity. As we saw, a biological learning process follows such recognition and culminates in immunological resistance.

Immunological recognition and external digestion are the artifices by which the biological self detoxifies foreign organisms and holds its ground. These two basic processes — *digestion* and *immunity* — are tied to different organic systems of the organism:

The 'I' with its constituent elements digests nutrients in the gastro-intestinal tract (external digestion). It transforms them into its own organic substance (internal digestion). This humoural build-up culminates in the blood. In this respect blood, as a humoural-cellular organ, is the direct bearer of the 'I'.

But the 'I' and its constituent elements also perceives invading foreign structures and develops specific actions to resist and reject foreign matter. It does this through the blood and lymphatic systems. The *lymphatic system*, again a cellular-humoural organ, serves the 'I' through immunological recognition and the development of immunological resistance.

CHAPTER FOUR

DIGESTION AND THE IMMUNOLOGICAL RECOGNITION OF FOREIGN MATTER

Digestion and immunological recognition —
polar actions of the metabolic system

We described earlier how the structure of the human 'I' in the metabolism engages in two basic functions: *digestion* and *the perception of foreign matter*. The digestive system processes the stream of nutritional substance in such a way as to allow the organism to build itself up humourally. In the first instance, this process culminates in the blood and leads to the organic self-representation of the individuality in the organism: the blood is the material vehicle of the 'I'. For the organism to build itself up from substance (nourishment) which is originally foreign, an artifice is required: rejection or decomposition of the alien form and ingestion of the substance. The nutritional *substance* can only be taken over by the biological self if it passes through an undifferentiated stage biologically or is already in that state from the beginning (e.g. water, glucose, etc.).[42]

The other action of the 'I' in the metabolism is the biological recognition of all foreign living matter which penetrates the organism by means other than the digestion (parenterally). This perception of foreign substance — primarily of the *form* taken by the substance, as with every perception — is directed specifically at the subtle structures of material particles which are present in minute quantities and dimensions. In the same way that digestion

---

42 Rudolf Steiner and Ita Wegman, *The Fundamentals of Therapy*, Chapter Eight.

assimilates the alien biological environment which the organism subsequently uses internally to build itself up, so the outward orientation of the biological self's resistance towards a hostile environment develops through perceptual activity by way of an unconscious biological learning process. The end result of digestion is thus the *construction of the self*; the end result of the perception of foreign matter is the *integrity* of the biological self. The medical term for this integrity is *immunity*.

Both nourishment and other foreign matter are *poison* to the organism. Why is the alien, the biological, non-self poisonous? The concept of poison as such is a relative one. A substance is always poisonous or non-poisonous only in relation to a biological organism. Therefore all substances whose structure has not been determined by the metabolic activity of the constituent elements of the organism, by the individual action of the 'I', or which cannot be integrated into that activity, are poisonous. Thus the organism continuously has to safeguard its biological territory through detoxification. This detoxification assumes the decomposition of the foreign matter: the substance has to be separated from its structure. This can be done in two ways: through digestion or perception. Digestion moulds the specific form of the self into the undifferentiated matter it has taken over. In a reversal of this process, immunological recognition incorporates the wealth of differentiated foreign forms into our organic structure.

The actions of the 'I' in the metabolism — digestion and immunological recognition — which we have described above, are polar activities. Nevertheless, they also work in close co-operation. This co-operation becomes more obvious when we take note of the following observation: on the one hand nourishment passes through a zone of — conscious — perception (smell, taste, touch) when it is first taken in, and only then does it pass into the digestive system; the latter culminates in the blood. On the other hand, the immunological processes start in all the tissues of the organism, become concentrated in the organs of the lymphatic system, and then lead into the subtle processes of parenteral digestion (i.e. occurring in all tissues and the blood), as will be shown in greater detail below.

These polar and yet closely interlinked actions of the 'I' come together in the organs of the integrated *tissue-lymph-blood system*. Since both actions are produced by a unified 'I' structure with its constituent elements — astral body, etheric body, physical body — the close morphological and functional links between the blood system and the lymphatic system is easy to understand. We will now look more closely at these latter two.

The blood and the biological individual between dispersion and self-perception

Blood is a fluid organ. Its cells — in contrast to the other organs — are not embedded in a colloidal or fibrous structure but are suspended in a fluid, extra-cellular substance. Only when the blood coagulates does it take on the colloidal-fibrous consistency which prevents it from spilling. The blood as a fluid (c.5 litres) only forms a unity when considered together with the vascular system; both are merely opposing expressions of the same organ-building impulse. This can be shown particularly clearly when we look at the embryological formation of the blood. The flowing plasticicity of the blood fluid can be directly grasped and penetrated by the etheric body. But the task of the vascular system can only be understood if the polar behaviour of the blood stream is taken into account. Its function spans both *dispersion* and *isolation*.

When blood flows to the periphery it issues through the *capillaries* and disperses in the tiny extra-cellular spaces which exist between the cells of the body; they are microscopically small in size but their total extent throughout the organism is so large that they can, for example, 'invisibly' hold ten litres of fluid. In this area the blood makes itself available to the organs and tissues, brings them nutrition and oxygen and washes away the waste products. It also serves to maintain body temperature. Blood 'cools' organs with a high temperature and 'warms' organs at a lower temperature.

Before and after this capillary section of the blood circulation

— i.e. in the arteries and veins — the blood is concerned only with itself, so to speak, and has no immediate functional contact with the other organs. This self-isolation of the blood reaches its greatest intensity in the heart. Many processes take place in this central organ of the blood circulation. We will note just one characteristic here. The *heart* is the organ where the blood encounters itself. For while the blood at the periphery flows into the differentiated sphere of the organs, penetrating them and washing through them down to the minutest level, it is concerned only with itself in the heart. The heart muscle is nothing more than a vascular organ of complex construction which has undergone further specific development, i.e. it is part of the structure which holds the fluid organ of the blood. The unbroken flow of the blood is stopped and 'apportioned' in the heart. For short periods at a time during the systole (when the valves are closed), the heart encloses a small portion of blood and thus experiences itself as it contracts — rather like the right hand can grasp and feel the left hand. An intensified process of self-perception lies at the heart of both cases. If we consider that this self-perception occurs in blood which has just concluded a motion of comprehensive diffusion throughout the organism, during which it has devoted itself to the variety of individual characteristics which make up the inner world of the organs while assimilating their very different traits, then this self-perception of the blood simultaneously incorporates an unconscious, comprehensive self-perception of the whole organism.

The motion of the blood thus alternates between diffusion and self-perception. The vascular system, mediating between the extremes of these two poles, participates in both actions: on the arterial side it takes care of the distribution of the blood into the infinitely spread-out, internal world of the organism, on the venous side it guides the blood to, and contracts it into, the heart.

In terms of 'complementary knowledge' [43], the above needs to be supplemented by a look at the supersensory human constituent elements. The etheric body enables the blood to flow through the

---

43 See Chapter One.

organism so that it returns to its starting point in a circular motion; for the etheric body lives in all regular, organic repetition. The action of the astral body is expressed in the alternation between diffusion and isolation, between distribution and concentration. The 'I' works in the blood as the central organ of homoeostasis, maintaining the overall balance between the individual aspects of the metabolism and the particular, localized organic structures. At any given moment the blood and its circulation establish the unity of the whole organism on a functional level, so that through this medium the 'I', from the inside, can turn the body into the bearer of identity, into a biological self.

The anatomical and histological structure of the blood circulation demonstrates — like no other system in the organism — a certain principle of construction. The division of the arterial vessels from the centre (heart) to the periphery (capillaries) guides the eye of the scientist beyond the point which marks the boundary between ordinary and microscopic visibility. For example, what appears to be uniform skin colour is revealed under the microscope to consist of a myriad of capillaries which — lying next to, but separated from, one another in finest loops — extend at the boundary of dermis and epidermis. At every moment the blood, as it flows through the organism, crosses the boundary between visible compactness (in the heart and the large vessels) and invisible microscopic structures. What the anatomist does artificially when he progresses from the macroscopic organ to its functional units and, indeed, the cells, by means of the microscope happens by natural means in the process of blood circulation. The blood itself 'microscopes' and 'macroscopes', as it were, as it circulates. If we could observe and experience the distribution of the blood it would appear to the naked eye as vaporization to invisibility on the one (arterial) hand and reconvergence to visibility on the other (venous) hand.

In Chapter One we described the microscopic examination of the organism as the view of a dimensional perspective which has the cell at its vanishing point. In its turn, the blood as a fluid organ is engaged in the rhythmically alternating passage from the macroscopic to the microscopic dimension and back again through its expansion to the periphery and concentration in the central organ. This means that there is a continuous transaction between the area primarily comprising the nervous and sensory system and that primarily of the metabolic system.

When a single cell is observed through the microscope, we *think* of this cell, in terms of complementary knowledge, as being embedded in the differentiated context of the whole human being, which includes the four constituent elements on a supersensory level. These four elements — both individually and as an overall structure — are pure action. They are engaged in their specific activities. These activities leave traces which are visible on a sensory level. They open the organism to sensory observation. If the supersensory activity leaves only fleeting traces which change rapidly, which show brief constancy of form, we are in the metabolic sphere of the organism. The cell is such a fleeting, rapidly changing, short-lived trace of a supersensory event. If the supersensory activity leaves more permanent, more clearly defined, more differentiated traces of the action of the etheric and astral bodies, we have before us on a sensory and visible level the human form in its hierarchical construction. We are now in the nervous and sensory sphere with our observation. Here the form is of relatively longer duration, as the supersensory elements do not intervene so actively to bring about change as they do with the cell. They have gradually withdrawn. But they can be recognized in the clearly formed trace they have left behind.

In other words, the morphological transition from the complex microscopic formations comprising the higher structures, which exist in the organs or the organism as a whole, to the elementary cell structures represents a progression from the nervous-sensory system to the metabolic and limb system, from the form pole to the substance pole. The metabolism as an invisible process is tied to fleeting, microscopically-sized structures. There is a reciprocal relationship between structure and metabolic motion: the simpler the form and the smaller the dimension, the more intense the metabolism in which the form is embedded.

A simple fact shows this strikingly. The metabolism of a cow weighing 500 kg produces approximately 0.5 kg of protein within twenty-four hours. 500 kg of yeast cells, on the other hand, can produce more than 50,000 kg of protein. The secret lies in the fact that the metabolic process is tied to the surface of the organic structures. If the surface area increases relative to the volume of a biological body the metabolic intensity increases by the same ratio. This law is connected with the surface/volume ratio. Geometrically: If a cube whose edges are 1 cm long is divided into cubes whose edges are 1 µ (0.001 mm) long, the result is 10^{12} cubes of 1 μ^3 each; the surface of these cubes is 10,000 times larger than the single cube. [44]

In sum, it has become evident that the cardio-vascular system of the blood is constructed on a threefold principle. The heart is the locus of the blood circulation where the blood is most strongly formed and the form most strongly concentrated. At the same time it is also the consciousness pole — an organ of perception. The heart is the 'head pole' of the blood circulation. The system develops its own metabolic segment in the capillaries. We have the rhythmical intermediary segment in the blood vessels, particularly the arterial ones. Here the arteries correspond to inhalation and the veins to exhalation.

The cardio-vascular system has to be understood as a self-contained 'subsidiary structure'. It lies in the nature of the organism to integrate a whole range of such subsidiary structures which are not connected arbitrarily but are related. Thus a subsidiary structure which is complete in itself is in turn integrated into the organism in a specific locality. On the one hand, therefore, it is a structure which represents the organism as a whole, but on the other hand it fulfils a subordinate, specific function in a given locus.

The threefold cardio-vascular system as a whole is situated in the total organism between rhythm and metabolism. That is why the heart participates in two functions. Along with the lungs, it is the rhythmical organ *per se* within the organism as a whole. In relation to the subsidiary structure of the organism described as the cardio-vascular system, it is the nervous and sensory system of this part of the human being.

---

44 Hans G. Schlegel, *Allgemeine Mikrobiologie*, Stuttgart 1985, p.11.

The lymphatic system — an organ of perception in the metabolism [45]

The lymphatic system is arranged in parallel to the blood circulation. But it accompanies only the venous and not the arterial side of the blood stream. Starting from fine, open fissures which form in the extra-cellular space of the tissues, the flow of lymph thickens into vessels whose walls gradually become stronger, and widen. Eventually they unite to form one of the numerous 'central organs' of the lymphatic system which are distributed throughout the organism, the lymph nodes. The lymph gathers along short pathways after having passed through the lymph nodes and finally enters the blood stream in the central section of the venous system below the heart. The way the lymphatic system is integrated into the organism simultaneously demonstrates its task. It does not participate in the motion of diffusion and vaporization on the arterial side of the blood circulation but, on the contrary, accompanies only the contracting side of the blood which leads to self-perception in the heart. It is a vascular system related to the veins and imitates the latter on a different level and with a different task until it reaches the central organ of the lymph nodes. The lymph nodes fulfil 'heart function', i.e. a perceptual function, in a certain sense. But the perception is not directed at the self — as with the blood in the heart — but at everything 'foreign' which penetrates the organism and its tissue and is subsequently transported to the perceptual organ of the lymph node. Physiologists describe the function of the lymph nodes as a 'filter' in the first instance; but they have increasingly discovered the greatly differentiated functions of these immunological organs of perception, recognition and defence to be very complex [46] (Diagram 7).

If we consider the function of the lymphatic system in the context of its proximity to the blood circulation, it can be seen

---

45 See Matthias Girke, "Die Idee der Dreigliederung in immunologischen und entzündlichen Reaktionen", in: *Beiträge zu einer Erweiterung der Heilkunst nach geisteswissenschaftlichen Erkenntnissen* 1/1986.

46 Johannes Rohen/Elke Lütjen-Drecoll, *Funktionelle Histologie*, Stuttgart/New York 1982. Chapter: "Lymphatische Organe und Immunsystem".

Diagram 7

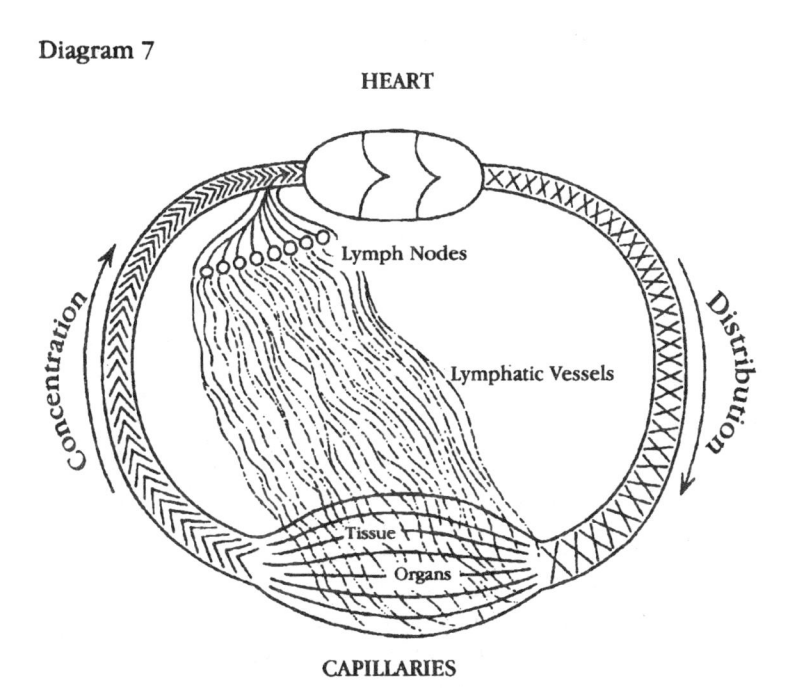

```
         HEART
    ↗              ↘
Concentration   Distribution
    Lymph Nodes
    Lymphatic Vessels
    Tissue
    Organs
       CAPILLARIES
```

that it serves subconscious perception through its connection with the venous aspect. But if we inquire after the position of the lymphatic system within the threefold context of the organism as a whole, we find that it is more deeply embedded in the metabolic sphere than the blood system. It is a part of the metabolic system, although a highly specific one. At the deep, unconscious level of the metabolism it conveys those processes of external or 'foreign' perception which human beings accomplish on a conscious level through sensory perception and its connected learning processes through the nervous and sensory system. In this sense the lymphatic system is a particularly developed cephalic organ embedded at the functional level of the unconscious metabolism.

The function of the lymph nodes as 'filtering organs' in the network of lymphatic vessels coming from all tissues is performed for the blood by the *spleen*. The latter, too, is an immunological organ of perception and resistance. Nevertheless, it does not fulfil that function in relation to the more outwardly directed boundaries of the organism (skin and mucous membrane) but in relation to the central organ of the blood itself. It is — among other functions — the 'frontier guard' for the human blood.

The cellular and humoural instruments of the immunological processes

The immunological processes, both cellular and humoural, reside initially in the blood. Blood cells, which account for 40 — 45% of the blood, originate in the bone marrow, the 'breeding ground' of the blood. By contrast, the fluid component of the blood is replenished all the time from nutritional fluid, flows through the blood vessels, tissues and organs, and is then continuously excreted (kidneys, breathing, skin). The c.7% protein contained in blood plasma originates in the cellular structural matter of the inner organs, e.g. the liver. Only certain cells and proteins in the blood are involved in the immunological processes. While the vast majority of all blood cells — the red blood cells — remain strictly within the vascular system and all carry out the same function, namely the transport of oxygen, all white blood cells (leucocytes) are able to leave the vascular system in order to carry out their function in other organs and tissues. The various types of white blood cells, which can be quite different from one another, are all concerned with maintaining the integrity of the organism in the face of an alien organism (immunity). We may note that these various populations of leucocytes range between the metabolic poles of digestion on the one hand and perception of foreign matter on the other, as discussed earlier.

Diagram 8

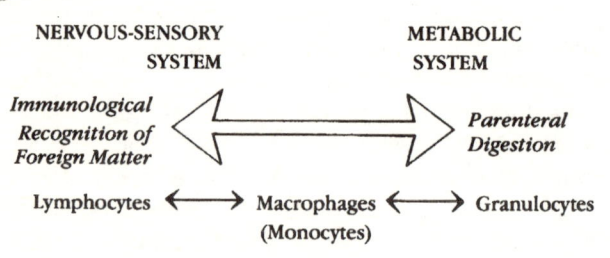

```
           NERVOUS-SENSORY              METABOLIC
               SYSTEM                    SYSTEM
      Immunological    ⟨⎯⎯⎯⎯⎯⎯⎯⎯⟩    Parenteral
      Recognition of                    Digestion
      Foreign Matter

         Lymphocytes ⟵⎯⎯⟶ Macrophages ⟵⎯⎯⟶ Granulocytes
                           (Monocytes)
```

There is a surprising variation in the life-span of the blood cells. While the red cells may live between 120 and 130 days, the leucocytes may live for between two to three days and several months, even years, depending on their character and function. The life-span is clearly connected with their respective function: *granulocytes*, which are the bearers of tissular digestive processes, belong to the short-lived leucocytes, while *lymphocytes*, which deal with immunological recognition of a nervous-sensory nature, live longer, some of them probably for a very long time. The *macrophages* represent a cell population some of which also originate in the blood stream (monocytes) and migrate to the tissue. There they are active in the digestive tissular metabolism as well as providing decisive support in the recognition of foreign matter by the lymphocytes.[47]

Processes of specific immunity [48,49]

The lymphocytes are the carriers of specific immunity, i.e. they are able to recognize a foreign agent which has infiltrated the organism by by-passing the regular digestive system (through the skin, the mucous membranes, the respiratory pathways, the gastro-intestinal tract, etc.) and to develop resistance against it. But this resistance is so specific that it matches only a particular agent, just as a given key only matches a given lock. The foreign agent is called an *antigen* in immunology and the defensive structure possessed by the organism is called an *antibody*. The key-lock principle applies strictly in all cases. Nevertheless, foreign matter, (bacteria, for example) often carries several antigenic determinants on its surface while the lymphocytes carry only one structural antibody. Since such

---

[47] The breadth and scope of scientific knowledge about all these functions is enormous. At the boundaries of this knowledge hypothetical assumptions and probabilities do, of course, arise. In the context of the anthropological approach with which we are concerned here, we can sketch out only a few of the most important facts.

[48] P.A. Berg/P.V. Lehmann, "Immunologie in der inneren Medizin", in: *Klinik der Gegenwart*, vol. II, 1984 version.

[49] Robert Keller, *Immunologie und Immunpathologie*, Stuttgart 1981.

one-off and specific key-lock relationships are called clones, one can say that lymphocytes are always monoclonal while many antigenic materials (including bacteria) are polyclonal.

Since specific immunity is something which is acquired during life, the infant organism develops a wealth of immunological responses during the course of childhood as a result of contact with the alien biological environment after birth. It has been calculated that c. 10^8 different clones are formed by the approximately 2×10^{12} lymphocytes present in the human organism.[46,48] This means that in the lymphocytes and the antibodies which they form we carry around with us an infinite amount of structural world-representation in material form. Such immunological world-representation has to be acquired after birth and is tied to the cell population of the lymphocytes. This acquisition also explains the initially high percentage of lymphocytes in the blood stream which is slowly reduced during the course of childhood until we reach adulthood. With a newborn child it amounts to c. 50 — 60%, while in adulthood it is no more than 20 — 25%.

Within the lymphocyte population there is once again a polar division in the direction of their activity. From their joint origin in the bone marrow, there is a divergent development in the population. One population, the T-lymphocytes, leaves the bone marrow via the blood and establishes itself in the thymus gland. This gland originates at the embryonic stage — like the thyroid gland — in the area of the pharyngeal pouches of the upper digestive tract and extends downwards in the middle of the chest behind the breastbone. It begins to regress in the course of childhood and youth and later atrophies altogether. The lymphocytes mature in this thymus gland, which is why they are called T-lymphocytes. When they are fully developed they return to the blood and are distributed throughout the organism, establishing themselves mainly in the lymph nodes and the spleen. But they are also found wherever the organism is in contact with the external environment (skin and mucous membrane). Another population of lymphocytes, called B-lymphocytes, remain in the bone marrow until maturity and then migrate and are distributed, like the T-lymphocytes, in the lymphatic organs described above, i.e. mainly in the lymph nodes and the spleen.

But neither type of lymphocyte remains resident solely in the lymphatic organs. They 'travel unceasingly through lymphatic tissues of the body with the aim of tracking down antigenic material. On their journey they always follow the same route: via the blood stream they enter the lymphatic organs, particularly the lymph nodes and the spleen, and from there they return to the blood stream via efferent lymphatics and the thoracic duct (main channel of the system of lymphatic vessels). Transportation through the blood vessels ensures the regular redistribution of the various lymphocytic clones to all the lymphatic regions of the body in which the encounter with antigens takes place.' [50]

It has been established that a lymphocyte completes this cycle in about 18 hours.

How do the lymphocytes activate recognition, memory and resistance? These cells only achieve their final functional maturity through contact with foreign antigenic structures. Only this perceptual contact, which takes place on the cell membrane, awakens the full vitality of the cell, its proliferation. Without this functional awakening the cell would die in a short space of time. At this point it develops a counter structure on its surface which corresponds exactly to the structural pattern of the foreign antigen, rather like a seal imprinting its image on the sealing wax. This clones the lymphocyte. The proliferation of these monoclonal T-lymphocytes develops in two different directions: the cytotoxic T-cells and the T-memory cells. When the former encounter foreign cells on their journey which correspond to the clone the foreign cells can be killed off. This is done through poisons which cytotoxic T-cells develop following primary contact. Such foreign cells to be killed off can include cells belonging to the organism itself which have been invaded, i.e. infected, by foreign antigens. The cytotoxic T-lymphocytes are short-lived. By contrast, the T-memory cells can be extremely long-lived under certain conditions. Their function is to preserve the clonal structure, and always 'remember' the primary contact whenever they have renewed encounters with antigenic structure on their travels. Their reaction consists of transformation into proliferating

---

[50] Berg/Lehmann, *op.cit.*

lymphoblasts — these are youthful forms of the cell — whose revived vitality and proliferation again produces cytotoxic and memory cells. The cycle repeats itself, but on a higher level insofar as the intensity of resistance and 'acquaintance' have remained from the earlier first contact.

As well as the two sub-populations of T-lymphocytes described above, there are others which we encounter in describing the B-lymphocytes. Here, too, contact with an antigen awakens the cell to become fully functional. This function, however, does not consist in the development of an anti-toxin which only works from cell to cell through direct contact, but in the development of so-called antibodies. These are proteins which are monoclonally structured but which are freely released by the B-lymphocytes into the tissue of the lymph nodes and from there into the blood stream. There they form part of the blood protein (immunoglobulin). They participate in many ways in the resistance against antigenic foreign matter. Above all, they enter a so-called antigen-antibody reaction with the foreign antigen and form an antigen-antibody complex (immune complex) which 'detoxifies' the antigen. This inactive material complex can then be fed into the parenteral digestion.

A third population of T-lymphocytes is involved in the process which transforms the B-lymphocytes into the antibody-forming B-lymphoblasts (plasma cells). These are the T-helper cells. Here we encounter the specific way in which immunological decisions are made. For both the T- and the B-lymphocytes do not react to simple contact with an antigen. There must always be simultaneous contact with a structure belonging to the biological self. 'Foreign' is only recognized in connection with 'own' or 'self' (dual recognition). The lymphocytes possess this highly differentiated type of recognition, which is modelled on the pattern of conscious judgement based on the interaction between world and self, between foreign and own. Thus B-lymphocytes can only be activated into transformation and antibody formation by an antigenic structure if they perceive contact with the organism's own structure *at the same time* as they perceive the antigen. This perceptual process is offered by the T-helper cells. Such structures, which are found on the cell membrane of the cells belonging to the organism itself and which represent the foreign antigen to every other organism, to every non-self, are called HLA antigens (a purely artificial term). Such HLA antigens are the markers by which the biological self recognizes itself. Thus T-helper cells assist the B-lymphocytes in recognizing foreign antigens. We can now ask what assists the T-lymphocytes in recognizing foreign structures? These are the macrophages. We will describe them further below, once we have dealt with non-specific immunity.

Non-specific cellular and humoural immunity

Non-specific immunity is phylogenetically older than specific immunity. That means that it is a more primitive, original way in which an organism defends itself against foreign matter and attempts to maintain its integrity.

Only the increasingly distinct way in which the biological individual develops in higher animals and, finally, in human beings allows a higher form of immunity, the specific immunity described above, to develop. As we saw, specific immunity makes use of the specific, deeply unconscious organs of consciousness, if I may be allowed that paradox. Immunological perception, memory, judgement and directed action can only be understood as a nervous-sensory activity in the unconscious metabolism. If we look at the nervous-sensory actions of the lymphocytes in connection with their particular characteristic of wandering through the organism as individual cells, we can understand how modern immunology refers to a 'mobile brain'.[51] Rudolf Steiner, too, describes this relationship between nerve cells and white blood cells — although he refers to it as a polar one.[52]

How does complementary knowledge conceptualize such a mobile organ? Apart from the sex cells of the human organism, there are no other cells which break away from the tissue except

---

51   J. Edwin Blalock/Eric M. Smith, 'The Immunesystem: our Mobile Brain', in: *Immunology today* 6, no.4, 1985.
52   Rudolf Steiner, *The Human Being in Body, Soul and Spirit*, lecture of 5 Aug. 1922. Rudolf Steiner Press, 1989.

the white blood cells, particularly the lymphocytes, which, as we saw, tour regularly around the organism. Since they do not belong to any physical organ — apart from their respective temporary residence in 'foster organs' — only the etheric body as supersensory life bearer and the 'I' with its associated biological judgement (astral body), are responsible for their co-ordinated action. Accordingly, the immunological organ is an extremely spiritual organ.

The cellular and humoural processes in *non-specific resistance* are completely different. The latter is considerably closer to the metabolic process and is therefore based largely on the many variations in, and forms of, digestion; this is represented archetypally in the gastro-intestinal tract but can be — parenterally — at work in metamorphosed form throughout the tissues and the organs. The processes of cellular resistance are tied to the polymorphonuclear leucocytes, above all the granulocytes. While the T- and B-lymphocytes are found mainly in the secondary lymphatic organs, the granulocytes are initially found mainly in the bone marrow and circulating blood. But with their enormous amoeboid motility they can immediately travel 'on call' from the blood to endangered areas of tissue if an acute invasion of foreign matter (infection) occurs there. Besides secreting numerous substances of toxic and digestive intensity into the tissue they possess, above all, the capacity for phagocytosis. The cell body flows around and engulfs the foreign matter, including mortified material from the organism itself, and digests it within the cell body (endophagocytosis). The cells belonging to this leucocyte population die off in the process and together these and the foreign matter form the pus which arises both in localized and in more extensive inflammations. Unlike the lymphocytes, this cell population therefore does not have the capacity to recognize foreign matter. It immediately goes over to the 'attack', to aggressive digestion, and can therefore strike 'friend and foe' equally. This 'blind' aggression, as it were, dangerous under certain circumstances, is only held in check because these cells do not become active unless 'called'. Such a summons is provoked by a number of factors in the change of environment in such areas of tissue where a foreign invasion has occurred (infection). The change in environment is primarily chemical, e.g. through strong acidification of the environment, but also occurs toxically (through bacterial toxins) or through lack of oxygen (due to interrupted blood flow). All these processes, which are only briefly indicated here, belong to the wider subject of inflammations, which will be dealt with in greater detail below.

The *macrophages*, which we have already mentioned, are also involved in non-specific cellular immunity. Functionally they are positioned between the lymphocytes and the polymorphonuclear leucocytes. In contrast to the lymphocytes, which are transported more passively and are washed to their area of function, the macrophages possess partial amoeboid motility — like the polymorphonuclear leucocytes. But while the latter have to be summoned in an 'emergency', most of the macrophages are settled to a greater or lesser degree in the tissue to which they have migrated from the blood (where they are called monocytes). In any case, they are not subject to the wanderings of the lymphocytes as they are spread throughout the organism. They keep a continuous watch in the tissue for foreign material and/ or degenerated material from the organism itself (cells or their remains, antigen/antibody complexes, etc.). They share the capacity for phagocytosis with the granulocytes and are therefore linked closely with digestion. They share the function of recognizing foreign matter with the lymphocytes, but unlike the latter they do not form monoclonal counter structures. This non-specific ability to recognize foreign matter is puzzling and no explanation has yet been found for it. The macrophages are long-lived, like the T-memory cells; they can persist in the tissue for months and years. Since the macrophages are involved in almost all processes of specific and non specific immunity their position and function can be seen as an intermediary one between the polar characteristics of digestion and recognition of foreign matter. They are indispensable to the integrity of the organic self since they provide the 'substructure' required by the highly specific cellular immunity.

Just as the whole organism is subject to a cellular and a humoural phase of activity, the functions of digestion and recognition of foreign matter also occur in cellular and humoural systems. But, most importantly, these systems work intensively together. They supplement each other to the extent that cellular activities can never become effective without humoural participation and vice versa. We have already seen how specific immunity begins as a cellular event but is then transformed into humoural activity with the formation of specific antibodies. In the field of non-specific immunity enzymes appear which may carry out a digestive function comparable to the digestive enzymes in the gastro-intestinal tract if they are activated by specific signals (the so-called complement system). These so-called mediators work more intensively and belong to the acute, indeed, most aggressive phase of humoural resistance. They are produced by certain sub-populations of the polymorphonuclear leucocytes and related cells in the tissue and are exceedingly aggressive. This shows once again the close links between cellular and humoural factors, particularly in non-specific immunity.

We cannot here go into all the details of this cellular-humoural interaction. It only needs to be remembered for the concluding section on allergies and inflammation that the more a metabolic process is connected with the parenteral digestion, the greater is the element of humoural activity. This is explained by the fact that digestion as such initially takes place largely in the amorphous humoural sphere. By contrast, the more a metabolic process is connected with the immunological recognition of foreign matter, the greater is the cellular participation in this action. Here, too, we are justified in referring to the organism as a whole: the sensory and nervous processes of conscious perception are based on structures which (in the sensory organs and the central nervous system) are practically exclusively of a cellular nature.

Allergies and inflammation — a polar relationship [53]

Parenteral digestion and immunological recognition can be described as actions of the whole organism, just like digestion and perception. All these actions belong to healthy processes in the organism and take place unnoticed, 'hidden'. Not so when

---

53 Cf. Volker Fintelmann, *Intuitive Medizin*, Stuttgart 1986.

the human being falls ill. Physiological activity then escalates beyond its normal, healthy levels. But this activity is also displaced and appears in areas of the organism where it is not normally at home (dislocations). Inflammations — of whatever type or location — can be understood as escalated and, above all, dislocated digestion. In contrast. the so-called allergic illnesses, from the chronic to the acutely critical ones, turn out to be excessive forms of resistance against foreign matter which have become established in the wrong place.

Two simple examples can demonstrate that: an infection occurs through a — not always medically clear — weakness in the inner assertiveness of the organism or through a powerful outside influence. If pneumonia develops, for example, what are the symptoms? Shivering fits and the ensuing high temperature show us a strong increase in the metabolic rate. The 'I' intervenes in the whole organism through the warmth body. In the lung the affected area is consecutively flooded, first humourally and then cellularly, with the biological instruments of non-specific resistance and escalated digestive power, as we have described. The initial humoural phase (serofibrinous inflammation) is followed by the cellular phase with the entry of blood cells into the air sacs of the lung. The granulocytes, summoned there en masse, kill the invading germs and form pus. Macrophages also appear at this point as these remains on the 'battlefield' of the inflammation are aspirated or coughed away. An accumulation of tissue, nodule-like and scar-like formations, can build up if the inflammation enters a chronic stage instead of healing immediately (e.g. with pulmonary tuberculosis). It contains increased numbers of lymphocytes. We can see that the instruments of the parenteral digestive forces of the organism are used in the feverish, hot beginning, but as the illness progresses the forces of immunological resistance are increasingly needed.

The reverse is the case with allergic processes. The most common allergy, particularly today, is hayfever, which is still on the increase in the population. The following happens with hayfever — as with other allergies: the antigen — in this case the protein-containing pollen of grasses, flowers or trees — provokes an immunological reaction on first contact in childhood. This, like most others, initially remains hidden. Antibodies have formed. Antibodies are still present, if in smaller numbers, at the next seasonal contact — i.e. one year later. But the memory cells have preserved the previous year's experience. Not immediately, but after a short latency period the first excessive symptoms of the allergy appear after contact with this year's pollen. Further contact later on can fuel the immunological reaction (booster effect). Hypersensitivity occurs. The symptoms can all be traced back to an excessive immunological reaction. In the case of hayfever they are initially restricted to the contact tissue: a strong, mostly runny cold with serous inflammation of the mucous membranes, reddening, itching, burning in the nose, the throat, the conjunctiva and eventually also the lower respiratory pathways. Fever occurs at the most intense level. In the case of other allergic illnesses the symptoms can spread throughout the whole organism (e.g. generalized allergic eczema of the skin).

The symptoms therefore show a polar relationship between allergy and inflammation. If, using the concepts of complementary knowledge, we try to understand this polarity by means of a conceptual threefold division of the organism, then both allergy and inflammation can be integrated into the threefold organism as a whole: immunological reactions start in the nervous and sensory system; they include the slow build-up of sensitivity which in full health remains without symptoms, 'hidden'. The increasing escalation of the allergic reaction, which can culminate in abrupt allergic shock following contact with an antigen (anaphylaxis), reveals an increasing intensity in the symptoms through to a generalized reaction: the whole organism becomes involved in the — under certain circumstances life-threatening — illness. The reverse development takes place with inflammations: they are typically highly acute and generalized (fever) at the beginning, then they subside and either normality is restored or they take a slow, mostly localized, chronic course.

These two initially separate pathological processes move in opposite directions both in relation to tempo and to the respective dominance of the threefold polarity. But allergy and inflammation cannot be separated: every process involving allergic illnesses uses inflammatory processes secondarily. Every inflammation develops immunological reactions as it runs its course. It follows from this conceptualization that a wealth of partly very complex forms of interaction between allergy and inflammation can occur in the pathological area extending between these two poles. In conclusion, we can show this context with a simple diagram:[54]

Diagram 9

Progression of immuno-reaction		Forms of immuno-reaction	Forms of inflam-mation		Progression of inflam-mation
	NERVOUS-SENSORY SYSTEM		NERVOUS-SENSORY SYSTEM		
Cellular field	T-Lymphocytes	Delayed immuno-reaction	Granulo-matous inflammation		Cellular field
	B-Lymphocytes	Immuno-complex reaction /	Chronic proliferative inflammation	Lymphocytes Macrophages	
Humoural field	Immuno-globulins	Cytotoxic immuno-reaction	Purulent inflammation	Granulocytes	Humoural field
	Complement Mediator substances	Immediate reaction	Fibrinous inflammation Serous inflammation	Complement Mediator substances	
	METABOLIC SYSTEM		METABOLIC SYSTEM		

The often quoted increase in allergic illnesses of all kinds rests without doubt in the specific circumstances produced by the living conditions in today's civilization. On the one hand there is an increase in industrial substances in the environment which place a great strain on the immune system. On the other hand our perceptual capacity is grossly overburdened. The systematic build-up of consciousness through perception, memory development, the formation of judgement and the

---

54 The diagram contained in the study by M. Girke (see note 45) is used here without alteration.

acquisition of skills is often steam-rollered by a profusion of stimuli. The phases become confused. This places a strain on the outwardly orientated experiential structures in the 'upper' human being: the upper astral body is increasingly drawn toward the environment (excarnated). This affects more than our consciousness (nervosity). At the same time the structures associated with the head also become organically oversensitive (allergies of the mucous membrane). The etheric body which controls the fluid in the organism follows this pull to the periphery and flows into the environment allergic runny cold [55]. This overloading makes it impossible for the 'I', which controls the relationship between the organism and its environment, between alien and self, to maintain the balance. The overwhelming of the human being by excessively powerful external influences on our perceptual processes in allergic illnesses thus has as its polar opposite the invasion by foreign matter of the digestive processes in inflammatory illnesses. In both cases — allergies and inflammations — the formative power of the organism in relation to external influences is fully intact; indeed, it is excessively active, developing some of its symptoms precisely for that reason.

In contrast, there are illnesses whose appearance is characterized by a weakness, indeed, by the total failure of the biological self in relation to the environment, which — as we saw — is always on the attack. AIDS, the Acquired Immunodeficiency Syndrome, and a source of great fear for people today, can be understood as such a failure of the biological self. The next three chapters will be devoted to a study of this illness on the basis of the knowledge of the human being which has been presented here.

---

[55] Cf. Steiner and Wegman, *op.cit.*, note 42.

CHAPTER FIVE

AIDS — THE DEADLY SEED

The new epidemic

The appearance of the new illness, AIDS, has been a surprise in two respects:
1. A new epidemic, against which there is initially complete therapeutic helplessness, has made its appearance among the populations of cities in advanced societies. This is a surprise above all because epidemics of this magnitude and of such an explosive nature were thought to have been eradicated by medicine, at least in developed countries.
2. The AIDS epidemic represents — and this is the second surprise — a completely new type of infectious disease. For the virus which causes the illness (HIV I; previously called HTLV III) does not primarily affect any organs, tissues or the organism as a whole, but specifically that biological system which is the carrier of resistance against infections, the centre of the immunological processes in the organism. That is also the reason why this illness is usually fatal. The AIDS patient does not die as a direct result of the infection by the virus but as a result of its consequences. AIDS merely clears the way for a multitude of other infections which spread unrestrained through the organism after the defences of the biological individual have been seriously damaged or destroyed.

When this epidemic appeared, medicine was sufficiently far developed to allow us to understand scientifically the cause and substratum of the pathological process in an astonishingly short period of time. This revealed that the focus of the infectious happening was the lymphocytes, that is, the carriers of specific immunity. This also explains the name of the illness: AIDS = Acquired Immunodeficiency Syndrome; similarly the pathogen: HIV = Human Immunodeficiency Virus.

On the one hand the epidemic gave immunologists confirmation of their astonishing research results and on the other it renewed their impetus. The illness presents researchers with an unplanned natural experiment of enormous magnitude.

But for anthroposophical medicine and its conceptualization of the human being AIDS represents a cognitive challenge of a different kind — quite apart from the question of therapy. We will attempt here to throw some light on AIDS from the point of view of spiritual science on the basis of the material we have previously considered.

The symptomatology of AIDS [56,57]

AIDS is a classic venereal disease with respect to the method of transmission. For if we disregard the artificial inoculation of the virus via the blood, sexual intercourse — both heterosexual and homosexual — remains almost the only natural means by which the virus can be transmitted. Beyond this, natural ways of infection also include the transmission of the virus from mother to unborn child through the placenta or at the time of delivery.

The inoculation of the virus occurs in a therapeutic context during the transfusion of blood or its components (stored blood and coagulation factors). It also occurs through the unhygienic or careless use of needles and syringes if the materials concerned are contaminated with the virus (drug addiction or medical use). The transmission of the virus through ordinary day-to-day social contact between people is highly unlikely according to the present state of knowledge.

The symptoms following infection can be observed in three stages during their slow development:

The *first stage* is thoroughly uncharacteristic and may sometimes even lack any symptoms at all. Flu-like symptoms and a slight

56 F. Schneit and K. Wolff (eds.), *AIDS*, Symposium, Vienna 1985; Vienna/New York 1985. E.B. Helm and W. Stille (eds.), AIDS, 2nd edition, Munich 1985.
57 E.B. Helm, W. Stille and E. Vanek (eds.), *AIDS*, annual conference of the German Society for Infectiology, May 1986; Munich/Berne/Vienna/San Francisco 1986.

feeling of illness may occur. Occasionally — as with flu — the nervous system may be affected with symptoms related to encephalitis or meningitis. This stage lasts from the first to the sixth week following infection *(clinical incubation period)* and subsides benignly. Weeks or years can pass between this first appearance and the second stage. The patient is clinically healthy and feels well during this more or less extended period of latency. Only the evidence of HIV antibodies marks him out as a (latent) AIDS patient. These antibodies only become evident in the blood six weeks after the infection or later, i.e. only following, or at the earliest, during the above mentioned temporary first symptoms. We now know that the period between infection, i.e. the appearance of the first symptoms of illness in the infected person and the evidence of antibodies in the blood can comprise a very long time, sometimes longer than six months. We may call this period the *serological incubation period*. In that respect alone AIDS is different from most other viral illnesses. Its incubation period, although variable, is of unusual length. If we take into account that during this comparatively long incubation period the danger already exists that the infected person may infect others, the uncertainty in the testing and use of blood preserves, for example, becomes clear. It is therefore impossible to be certain that blood preserves are uninfected in any given case.

Following the latency period, which can last months or years, the illness enters its *second stage*. This is generally called the lymphadenopathy syndrome (LAS). It is a swelling of the lymph nodes in various regions, but in at least two places. It can also occur as generalized swelling. This is supplemented by non-specific symptoms, i.e. symptoms of a general nature, such as night sweating, fever, diarrhoea, general weakness and weight loss. The patient feels, and is, ill. This stage, in turn, can last several years without any great change or with only minimal deterioration.

At any time within this second stage the *third stage*, so-called full-blown AIDS, can develop from the lymphadenopathy syndrome. The immune system has broken down completely and there is nothing to stop the entry and spread of pathogens of every kind (so-called opportunistic infections). Once this third stage, full-blown AIDS, has developed, 95% of all patients die within three years. Remission through a return to the second or even the first stage, either spontaneously or through treatment, has never been observed. If we take into consideration that there is also no record to date of a remission from the second to the first symptomless stage, the fatal outcome of the illness is only a matter of time, even for patients with the lymphadenopathy syndrome. Current research allows us to assume with some certainty that statistically there are ten lymphadenopathy patients and one hundred infected people not showing any symptoms for every patient with full-blown AIDS.

The symptoms of full-blown AIDS include, above all, three less frequently observed areas of illness:

1. A range of *infections* occur in an individual patient or in several patients, which appear in organs locally or regionally. These infections are called opportunistic. This indicates that any given pathogen which happens to encounter the organism is able to trigger an infection. Here we may observe that this occurs precisely with those pathogens which are otherwise rarely or relatively rarely infectious in non-immunodeficient people. They include *Pneumocystis carinii, Toxoplasma gondii, Cryptosporidium, Cytomegalovirus* and others. The pathogens which exist on and in the organism — also partially in the form of so-called saprophytes, as harmless, non-pathogenic inhabitants of higher organisms — now start to spread, giving rise to a variety of symptoms. These rare pathogens are not the only ones which gain ground in the conditions created by an immuno-deficient environment. Better known microbes such as the tuberculosis bacteria do the same. One of the most frequent opportunistic infections is — according to current reports — the form of pneumonia caused by the protozoan *Pneumocystis carinii* (with 80% of AIDS patients).

The opportunistic infections which appear with AIDS demonstrate by natural means something which can also be learned through a general study of the human being: throughout its life, the organism, the biological self, wages a 'positional war' at the boundaries of its immunological territory. At these boundaries 'alien' is perceived and judged to be 'non-self' in relation to 'self'. Effective defences are then erected and activated against this foreign non-self of the natural environment. But AIDS also demonstrates something in a practical way which would otherwise only be the subject of abstract, scientific research: microbiology shows that the whole of the environment which human beings inhabit is a place where myriads of invisible micro-organisms live. They populate not only the upper solid layers and the watery part of the earth's surface (hydrosphere) but are also present throughout the gaseous envelope of the earth (atmosphere) to a surprising height. Their distribution is extremely varied. Living in an unstable ecological equilibrium, they colonize — unseen but very effectively — specific sites. These frequently extend beyond inanimate nature into the biological interior of the higher animal and human organisms.

Thus there are bacteria in the human organism which penetrate deeply (the intestine, for example) into the area of the upper and lower orifices of the body and form colonies at the boundary of the human immunological territory. Here they live partially in a metabolic symbiosis with human beings, i.e. the vital processes of the intestinal bacteria and of human beings interact beneficially. While bacteria essentially live in dead or semi-dead matter (humus), which nevertheless extends into higher organisms like an ecological niche, viruses fundamentally require an organic, living environment to exist and multiply. Again and again micro-organisms invade the territory of human self-representation. After an initial conflict with the immune system, which may result in an inflammation, for example, these organisms can remain in a chronically adjusted state of equilibrium without having been completely killed and digested. This can happen with the *Mycobacteria tuberculosis*, for example, but also with the toxoplasmosis pathogens.

The biological self and the foreign nature of these micro-organisms maintain an — apparently motionless — equilibrium between them. But AIDS, in particular, demonstrates that this equilibrium is not a static one but an equilibrium of forces. The boundary between the biological self and foreign micro-organisms is therefore not only spacio-anatomical but essentially a dynamic one. It is present throughout the organism as an invisible boundary of forces. AIDS in particular shows that this equilibrium is not static and final: the disturbance of the state of equilibrium by this immunodeficiency illness results in secondary diseases in the form of inflammatory organic infections which are caused by the multitude of micro-organisms which colonize the boundary of the immunological territory.

It is immediately evident from the symptoms and the progression of the AIDS disease that the *biological individual is affected at the heart of his physical organic activity*. AIDS, then, does not strike at a more or less important organ whose function can be dispensed with or replaced, but at the core of the biological embodiment of the individuality, at the blood and lymphatic system.

2. A specific complex of symptoms affects the central nervous system. Besides the inflammations due to opportunistic pathogens which happen to affect the brain (e.g. *Toxoplasma gondii* and *Cytomegalovirus*), symptoms can be observed which are described as AIDS encephalopathy (brain disease caused by AIDS). It is found in approximately one third of patients with full-blown AIDS. If we include cases in which the symptoms are clinically absent but are shown to exist following autopsy, the nervous system is affected in 80% of patients with full-blown AIDS. The indications of a 'smouldering' change in personality with loss of strength and drive, paralysis of the emotional involvement in others' and one's own situation stand in the foreground. Patients give the impression of 'disinterestedness, slowing down, listlessness and apathy'. [57] Disorders of the mental processes (cognitive loss) also occur, resulting in increasing mental impairment and dementia due to organic brain disease. Some patients, indeed, develop regional failures of the nervous system — paralysis and absence of feeling.

The cause of all these symptoms must be sought in a special relationship between the HIV virus and the cells of the central nervous system. This neurotropism of the HIV virus causes the specific destruction of the brain. The dual relationship between the virus and the lymphocytes on the one hand, and the cells of the central nervous system on the other, comes as no great surprise. In Chapter Four we described the immune system as a cerebral structure in the metabolism. In addition, we came across the term 'mobile brain' used by immunologists to describe the population of lymphocytes with special perceptual abilities which travel through the organism. Thus the AIDS virus has an identical relationship with the two specific forms of perceptual cell structures: the 'mobile' cell system on the one hand and the fixed cell system of the central nervous system on the other. These two tropisms also largely determine the symptoms of AIDS through the diseases to which they give rise.

3. A third group of independent pathological processes in full-blown AIDS takes the form of certain tumours. It is not surprising that tumours occur in organisms from which the biological individual is expelled or withdraws because of illness. The more or less unrestrained spread of foreign matter in such an organism is indeed closely connected with the equally unrestrained spread of the organic cells of the organism itself. These, too, can withdraw — this is shown by the pathology of tumours — from the control of the biological individual and lead an independent existence in the organism as a foreign cellular sub-structure. All cancerous illnesses reveal something which is kept hidden in health: the continuous struggle of the human individual with the cellular part of the organism, which has the tendency to break out of the organism as a whole at any given moment and unfold its primitive individual characteristics. The conditions for such a 'break out' are created by AIDS and cause the organism to be flooded not only by foreign biological organisms from the environment, but by the cellular stock of the organism itself. The most important manifestation of cancerous illnesses in AIDS is *Kaposi's sarcoma*, a malignant vascular tumour which appears in the form of purple patches on the skin. It also includes certain lymphoma in the brain and elsewhere.

AIDS — a venereal disease

There is general agreement that AIDS is a new form of venereal disease. That does not mean that it is a disease which exclusively or primarily affects the sexual organs, but refers to the way in which it is transmitted, i.e sexual intercourse as the natural method of transmission of the pathogenic agent, the HIV virus.

The description of AIDS as a venereal disease is confirmed epidemiologically in that the spread of the illness appeared initially to be linked with homosexual groups around the world. The spread of the virus is not promoted by homosexuality as such but by the more widespread promiscuity among this group, that is, the more frequent change of sexual partner, than among heterosexuals, and this continues to be the case. From a radical utopian point of view, there is no doubt that the abstention from sexual intercourse, or at least strict monogamy, would eradicate AIDS within a few years. In this sense AIDS is a venereal disease (if we ignore the artificial methods of inoculation already mentioned above).

But there is an additional, extended sense in which this is the case from an anthroposophical point of view. An examination of the human sexual organization is necessary to make this clear. Such sexual organization represents a sub-structure of the overall organism — as we have already seen with other sub-structures — which has a threefold structure. These dynamic and morphological relationships have already been discussed. [58]

Such connections between the organism as a whole and the sub-organization of the 'sexual human being' will be developed here as far as is necessary. In order to do this, we have to use the preceding account of the threefold structure of the human organism as our immediate starting point (Chapter Three).

The threefold structure and sexual organization

The threefold organization encompasses the head pole and the limb pole, as well as the mediating rhythmical system. At the head pole the structure reaches the climax of its development — from a gross morphological point of view — in the formation of enclosed internal space. In a polar development, the organization is externalized in the limbs to such an extent that, far removed from its internal nature, it can intervene in its environment. On the basis of this polarity we can see that the human organism as a whole combines the fundamental characteristics of the female and the male elements:

The head as the pole of human self-unawareness has a receptive relationship to the world. It offers the perceptual impressions an

58 Klaus Dumke, 'Erkennen und Zeugen, Beitrag zu einer Menschenkunde der Geschlechter', in: *die Drei*, 9/1973.

internal space in which they can appear as such. Human beings subordinate themselves to external impressions at the head pole (subordinating pole) and form conscious ideas from them. This is not the case in the polar area of the limbs. Their outreach is an indication of the male character which actively intervenes in the world. In contrast to the internalizing gesture of the head cavity the limbs externalize the human form by aggressively reaching for the world (force or aggression pole). The cardio-pulmonary sphere forms the boundary between the external environment internalized through the senses and the power of the 'I' anchored in the blood, between the environmentally-orientated organs of the nervous and sensory system (head) and the self-orientated organs of the metabolic and limb system. In the heart we encounter the representation of the archetypal male-female form (hermaphrodite) which precedes all polarities between the sexes and which conciliates between them. The rhythmical intermediary function of the heart between head and abdomen can be demonstrated morphologically and physiologically in many ways. We will indicate only one morphological feature here: The central nervous system and the sensory organs are organized strictly in pairs; the digestive system, in contrast, is not. The heart, in its very complex embryological development, shows the intimate meshing of the paired, bilaterally symmetrical and the unpaired principle of construction.[59] It is exactly situated in the rhythm-providing centre between top and bottom, between world-orientation and self-orientation.

The complete human being is both male and female in organization, and contains the tendencies inherent in both. This enables an individual to be the instrument of incarnation of a being, a spiritual individuality, whose activity takes place beyond either the female or male character. But as a complete organism the human being cannot produce descendants; for that he needs the specific organization of the reproductive organs. The sexual organs are seated in the sphere of the metabolic and limb system. They are thus under the influence of the pole of motion, life and regeneration, and their activity takes place largely unconsciously. The place where

---

[59] Thomas Göbel, 'Das Herz als Stauorgan', in: *Mitteilungen des C.G. Carus-Instituts*, No. 47/1983.

human beings incessantly build up, regenerate and preserve their own bodies ('self-representation') through the incessant activity of digestion and reconstruction of matter, must undoubtedly also be the location for the structure which creates a totally new body: for reproduction. Here the female sexual organs are situated to a great extent in the internal spaces of the body, i.e. in the metabolic zone, for they fulfil a receptive, protective function. The male sexual organs, by comparison, belong spatially more to the lower limbs; their function is actively directed outwards like the limbs.

The anatomy of the sexual organs has — like the whole human being — a threefold structure. [60] But this threefold structure is organized in a polar fashion because of the polarity of the sexes. Ovaries and testicles are bilaterally symmetrical, like the nervous system, and the organs primarily under its influence. Both — like the nerve pole — are round. They essentially perform a dual function:

1. The primary task of the gonads includes their incretory functions. They establish hormonal control in the reproductive processes and beyond that exercise a fundamental formative influence on the development of the organism (primary and secondary sexual characteristics). This shows them to be related to the head pole in so far as they exert a controlling and formative influence, although differing inasmuch as this influence is not exercised throughout the organism by way of the nerves, but uses intermediary substances (hormones) in accordance with the siting of these organs deep down in the metabolic sphere.

2. Besides these primary controlling and formative tasks, ovaries and testicles also perform certain 'fostering services'. As embryologists have known for a long time, the male and female sex cells by no means originate in these organs. [61] On the contrary, they migrate to these 'fostering organs' through their amoeboid motility at a very early stage of embryonic development. They remain there for a long time until they reach full functional maturity, but they leave them again once they have attained that stage. Thus they

---

60 Paul Paede, 'Die Fortpflanzungsorgane des Menschen und ihre Spiegelbereiche', in: *Ärzte-Rundbriefe der Arbeitsgemeinschaft Anthroposophischer Ärzte,* Nos. 9 — 10/1949.
61 Dietrich Starck, *Embryologie,* Stuttgart 1965.

represent a cell system which, although settled for a long time, is fundamentally mobile. The target of their functional maturity is attained when they give up any links with the organism in which they originate, which for the male spermatozoa involves leaving the organism of origin altogether. The female ovum becomes independent in this way at the moment of ovulation. As solitary cells (functional unicellular organisms), the achievement of their functional aim — fertilization — coincides, both for the ovum and the sperm, with the almost complete loss of vitality. [62] Death of the sex cells or fertilization — that is the alternative for both structures when they reach the height of their maturity.

The specific nature of the motility of this sexually polarized cell system contrast greatly with the cell clusters which are otherwise found in organs and tissues, with one exception: the white blood cells. As we saw earlier, they also represent a mobile cell system. The lymphocytes are transported rather more passively through the system, while the granulocytes in contrast move actively from the blood into the tissues. In this respect they can be compared to the passive transportation of the ova on the one hand, and the active movement of the sperm cells on the other. In the same way that the sex cells mature in foster organs, the lymphocytes also inhabit such an organ, the thymus, for a time and leave it as they achieve full functionality. There can be no doubt that there is a close *affinity between the system of the immunocytes and the sex cells*. We need to examine this affinity more closely.

Within the threefold nature of the sexual organs, the female vagina and the male penis represent, in their anatomical complementarity, aspects of the limb and metabolic system. The non-paired structure of vagina and penis indicate that they belong to the organs of the metabolic system. But there is one peculiarity: the internal pairing of the upper erectile tissue in the penis indicates a hidden relationship with the paired limbs.[60] The vagina is a rudimentary hollow organ, as it were, while the penis is a rudimentary limb. The female organ, then, belongs to a greater extent to the internal organization of the abdominal cavity, the male organ to a greater extent to the external organization of the limbs. The latter

62 Johannes Rohen and Elke Lütjen-Drecoll, *Funktionelle Histologie*, Stuttgart/New York 1982.

even affects the testicles, which in the later stages of embryonic development descend from the protection of the abdominal cavity. Indeed, the functional ability of the testicles is tied to this limb-like tendency as they descend.

The head-orientated organs (ovaries and testicles) and the metabolic and limb organs (vagina and penis) within the reproductive system are separated in women by the womb as the mediating, rhythmical organ. Here the same formative and functional impulse which is found in the heart in the organism as a whole is realized on a more primitive, metabolic level. Like the heart, the womb develops embryonically from the symmetrical combination of a pair of ducts (paramesonephric or Müllerian ducts). Their spiral muscular construction can be directly compared with the heart. In the uterus, the female organism develops a centrally located predominant organ, whose function is organized in a strongly rhythmical way (menstrual cycle). The corresponding organ in men, the male uterus, is highly rudimentary. In this sense the male sexual organs are sharply polarized between the pronounced head organs (testicles) and the limb organization (penis).

We cannot, in this context, deal with our understanding of the psychological situation of men and women and the differing shaping of consciousness which follows from what we have just discussed. More on this can be found in the study mentioned earlier.[58] Next, we will consider separately the interaction of the sexes on a cellular level with respect to fertilization.

Fertilization — identity of perception and digestion

The fertilization of the female by the male sex cell represents in each case an absolutely solitary process in the life of metazoic (multi-cellular) organisms. It is cell division — and thus multiplication — which generally only occurs in the life of these organisms, whereas fertilization results in unification and thus, initially, a reduction in numbers. The reverse of the 'normal' functional direction which is found in fertilization also extends to the nuclear substance of the cell. As we shall see, nuclear substance normally migrates only from the nucleus to the body of the cell, but in fertilization it migrates 'backwards' from the body of the cell to the nucleus. This unique process of reversal of the 'normal' course of events characterizes the difference between sexual and asexual reproduction.

A second characteristic of sexual reproduction, which differentiates the latter from other biological processes involved in the continuous regeneration of metazoic organisms, is the following: in fertilization a structure which is alien to the female organism — the male sperm cell — is introduced into the territory of the biological self and united with the female egg cell. As we saw earlier, a comparable process takes place in the immunological processes. In the latter, matter invades the organism from the outside, is perceived as 'alien' by the immune system and detoxified as resistance is set up (the so-called immune complex), before finally being fed to the parenteral digestion (outside the gastro-intestinal tract).

In view of these immunological processes, the question arises as to whether a similar process takes place in fertilization. Here, too, we would expect to see perception of foreign matter (toxins), followed by detoxification through the formation of complexes, with the subsequent digestion of the alien structure which has been fixed in the complex. Is this expectation confirmed when we look at fertilization?

In the first instance the immunological processes take place essentially on the surface of the cell, the *cell membrane*. It is the sensitive organ of perception for the immunological recognition of alien matter (so-called membrane receptors). This perception — as we saw earlier — affects the whole cell. The lymphocytes react by proliferating, i.e. by 'waking' from their dormant state of perception into a state of active cell division. Thus, approximately 1000 daughter cells can develop from a single lymphocyte in a short period of time, all of which belong to a clone.[63] The immunological anti-bodies to any such perceived alien structures are therefore considerably multiplied through such cell division.

With fertilization, on the other hand, the 'perception' of the alien structure takes place in the *cell nucleus* itself. The alien structure which is perceived is not a bacterial envelope, a viral

63 Robert C. Gallo, 'Das Aids-Virus', in: *Spektrum der Wissenschaft*, 3/1987.

envelope or a viral capsule, all of which form protein-containing structures, but the genome of the spermatozoon itself. This genome — like that of all cells — consists of a protein-free substance which possesses an entirely individual structure. The immunological processes show that immunological recognition requires the preparation of receptors which have to fit the antigen like a key fits the lock.

Similar preparation is found in sexual recognition (= fertilization) although in a different way. The reduction divisions which introduce the final perceptual maturity of the male and female gametes are nothing other than the preparation of these cells for fertilization. The genome structure of both cells is halved in the process (haploid cells). This gives one cell the negative form which the counter-structure of the other can latch on to. During fertilization the female negative form is completed by the male positive form — or conversely, the male negative form by the female positive form — to introduce the diploid phase. And just as detoxification is the result of such a linkage between 'self' and 'non-self' in the immune complex, this also occurs in fertilization. For the sexual process as such is, in the first instance, a highly toxic one. 'It must be clearly understood that the human organism is indeed a completely self-contained system and that everything which lies outside it is, to a greater or lesser degree, toxic. Everything, then, which lies outside the human organism is poison. But there is a certain process of adaption which isolates, as it were, the otherwise poisonous effects. And this isolation of an effect which is poisonous in other circumstances appears ... specifically when the female and male seeds combine. It happens in many other cases as well, but particularly when the female and male seeds combine. The effect is exceedingly poisonous when these two opposing substances combine.' [64]

Why is this effect 'exceedingly poisonous'? The processes by which the sex cells — both male and female — reach maturity lead to the 'isolation' of these cells from their organic surroundings. This isolation also explains why test-tube fertilization is possible. The cells are isolated from the surrounding tissue and, lastly,

---

64 Rudolf Steiner, *Physiologisch — Therapeutisches auf Grundlage der Geisteswissenschaft. Zur Therapie und Hygiene* (GA 314), (Fundamentals of Anthroposophical Medicine), Dornach 1975, lecture of 2 January 1924.

the surrounding supersensory elements of the male and female organism. They are no longer part of the domain of the biological self. They are 'outlawed' as it were. In this sense the fertilization process is not an encounter of 'self' and 'alien', as in the immunological processes, but of 'alien' and 'alien'. This makes it 'exceedingly poisonous', for the effect of foreign matter is toxic.

Diagram 10

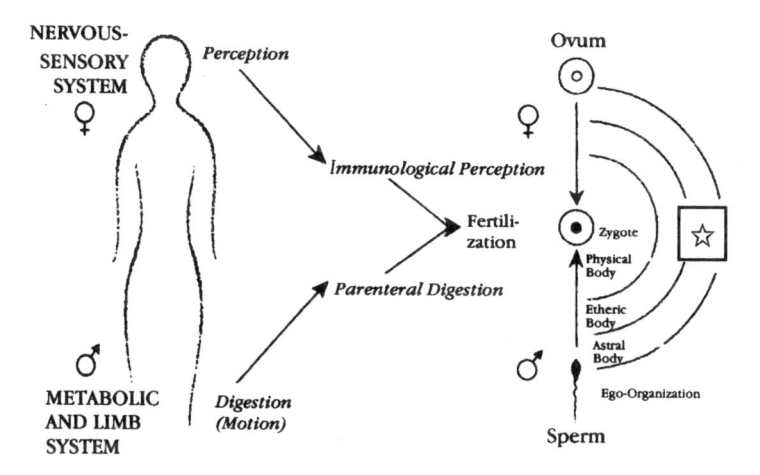

```
NERVOUS-SENSORY SYSTEM ♀         Perception              Ovum ♀
                                                          ○
                          Immunological Perception
                                                    Fertili-  ● Zygote
                                                    zation    ┃ Physical Body
                          Parenteral Digestion                 ┃ Etheric Body
                                                               ┃ Astral Body
METABOLIC                                              ♂       Ego-Organization
AND LIMB          Digestion                         Sperm
SYSTEM ♂          (Motion)
```

| ☆ | The supersensible human being at the beginning of Incarnation
Primal Perception
Primal Digestion |

But if the sexual complex which is thus formed were merely isolated it would die. And that, *de facto*, frequently happens. But if fertilization takes place, the following occurs: the process of encounter between the gametes, which have been isolated from the male and female organism, takes place because of the isolation described above. That means it is affected by cosmic forces and not — as with the immunological processes — the forces of the biological self. The sexual complex is 'exposed' to the forces of the world: 'The effect is an exceedingly poisonous one, but it is isolated, and through that isolation exposed to the forces of the cosmos, which can be described in detail'. [64] This initial action occurs in the context of the activity of a supersensory organism — that of the incarnating child. And the elements which comprise the supersensory being of the child are composed by specific cosmic forces. We can also describe this initial action as nutrition; i.e. the nourishment of the incarnating human being begins with the assimilation of the zygote into the supersensory human being (primal nourishment).[65] The generation of a new life begins at this point. In this respect the subsequent attachment (nidation) of the fertilized egg cell to the lining of the womb is secondary and — in view of the birth later on — temporary. For the second time the egg cell now inhabits a foster organ, the womb.

In summary, it can be seen that the fertilization process is very closely connected to the immunological process. The lymphocytes develop — like the sex cells — to full maturity in a foster organ, i.e. they develop the ability to perceive 'foreign' matter. They die off if, shortly after maturity, they do not encounter a foreign structure as they wander through the organism, and thereby become cloned. Similarly, ovum and sperm die off immediately if there is no encounter, i.e. fertilization. If the encounter takes place, if an immune complex or a sexual complex (zygote) is formed, the cell does not die but actively proliferates. The immunological cells incorporate a tremendous amount of outside information into the organism of the carrier; equally the developing zygote contains outside information from both the male and female elements. The zygote, in turn, is the starting point for the infinite number of somatic cells of the developing organism, in whose genomes the two complementary structures are present as a diploid genetic complex. The supersensory elements of the child incorporate the zygote into their overall activity and penetrate it as their instrument of incarnation in the same way that the immune complex is digested in the parenteral metabolism after detoxification. And just as the immunological information about the external environment serves the biological self as an instrument of defence against an alien environment, so is the cellular self-representation, the individual make-up of the infant organism, formed from the sexual complex.

If we bear in mind that the whole organism is male-female in construction, that sexual organization then develops either to the male or female pole on the basis of this male-female foundation, we

65 Cf. Chapter Two.

can expect to see renewed harmonization of the threefold structure when fertilization — which unites what is divided — occurs. Our investigation has shown that fertilization is indeed a process in which perception and digestion, the two basic processes of the polar organism, meet directly. This harmony creates an organic territory which can be used by a spiritual individuality as the field of activity for its incarnation. It is, after all, this individuality which perceives and takes possession, which digests.

AIDS — a diseased fertilization

Our earlier study of the threefold nature of the sexes pursued the initial question as to whether some light could be thrown from this perspective on AIDS as a new venereal disease. It can now be answered.

AIDS is a viral illness. How should viruses be characterized in the context of the forms and forces of nature? [66] Viruses can be understood as one-sidedly developed forms in the realm of micro-organisms. The micro-world can essentially be divided into unicellular organisms, bacteria and viruses. The *unicellular organisms* are differentiated from bacteria and viruses primarily by the fact that they are the most primitive living entities in which a trace of the threefold structure of organisms can still be recognized.[67] They are also the smallest independently living sub-structure through which stage the human organism physically passes in its development.[68] The nucleus with its surrounding membrane can be clearly recognized in the protoplasm which in turn is surrounded by an outer membrane (cell membrane).

In the protoplasm we have before us the intensive infinity of never-ceasing metabolic activity. It is tied to protein as the basic substance of life. In contrast, the specific configuration of the structure-giving and direction-giving genome of the cell is concentrated in the nucleus. The cell body forms the pole of metabolic motion while the nucleus provides the form pole.

---

66 This question will also be further dealt with in Chapter Six.
67 Ernst Wiesmann et al, *Medizinische Mikrobiologie*, Stuttgart/New York 1986.
68 Cf. Rohen/Lütjen-Drecoll, loc.cit., note 62.

Although the nucleus does contain protein, the structural information is tied to a non-protein substance, the nucleic acids. These are carriers of the very individually formed micro-configurations which represent the information pertaining to the organism on a material level.

A series of further facilities in the cell, which are anatomically fleeting but functionally all the more active, represent its transportation and respiratory system. This acts as an intermediary between the nucleus and the cytoplasm as well as between the interior and the exterior of the cell. But the information contained in the nucleus does not remain at rest there either. It is filtered into the plasma from the nucleus in the form of nucleic acid. The metabolic processes in the cell body could assume any form and develop in any direction in the infinity of possible motions, and the elements which are filtered out of the information centre give clear instructions as to the direction of the metabolic motion and its pattern. During this process the nuclear substance, which consists chemically of deoxyribonucleic acid (DNA), is copied so that its fine structure is replicated identically to form ribonucleic acid (RNA). It is the RNA which leaves the nucleus as copied information and gives instructions to the formative metabolic processes. The RNA therefore performs a messenger function between the nucleus and cytoplasm (messenger RNA).

Such cells, which still give a full indication of the threefold structure of organic matter, are called eukaryots. Their nucleus is clearly separated from the cytoplasm by a membrane.

Bacteria and viruses no longer conform to the harmonious threefold structure of life on a micro-level. On the contrary, *bacteria* and their life processes are best understood if they are conceived of as an infinite multiplication of cell bodies, as roaming metabolic systems. They do not possess a nucleus, or at most, primitive forms (or fragments) of one. That is why they are called prokaryots. Their source of information, i.e. the DNA structures which give direction to the metabolism, are scattered throughout the cell body whose immense metabolic productivity predominates. The imbalance between the strength of the metabolic motion and the much less developed informational

AIDS — THE DEADLY SEED

Diagram 11

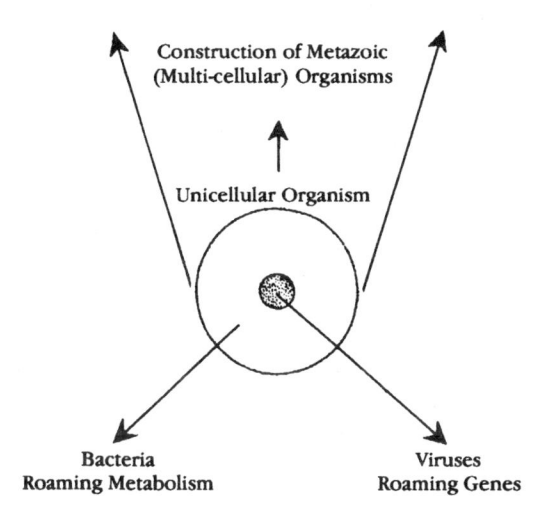

```
              Construction of Metazoic
              (Multi-cellular) Organisms
                        ↑
              Unicellular Organism
                    (○)
         ↙                        ↘
    Bacteria                     Viruses
    Roaming Metabolism           Roaming Genes
```

constancy also results in the great capacity for variance in the bacterial metabolism.

The *viruses* are completely different. They can be thought of as nuclear matter which has been removed from the harmoniously balanced whole of the cell (whereby this is not intended as any kind of theory of their factual genetic origins).

Viruses are freely 'roaming genes' [67,69], i.e. the material carriers of a constant configuration of information. They do not have a metabolism of their own so they are not actually living organisms. They do not reproduce autonomously but multiply through living substances, i.e. through cells and their metabolic activity. To use an extreme description, bacteria are 'roaming stomachs', viruses are 'roaming heads', if we take the cell nucleus with its genome as the 'head' and the cytoplasm with its metabolism as the 'stomach' of the cell.

There are various ways and means by which viruses multiply in living cells. These are dependent on the nature of the genome, that is, the encapsulated matter which holds the genetic information. There are DNA viruses, whose genome contains nucleic acid

---

69 Bruce Alberts, M. Raff et al, *Molekularbiologie der Zelle*, Weinheim 1986.

of the type found in the nucleus of eukaryotes. The RNA viruses contain a genome whose substance corresponds to the messenger RNA of the cell body. When viruses multiply, the viral DNA which has been introduced into the cell is built into the genome of the host cell and is replicated in and/or with its nucleus when it divides. By contrast, the RNA of the RNA viruses is replicated in the cell body in the same way as the messenger RNA. The DNA viruses are thus related more to the 'head pole' of the host cell, the RNA viruses more to the 'metabolic pole'.

But a peculiar type of virus is related to both poles: the retrovirus. After their genome has been introduced into the cell body, these RNA viruses initially undergo a transformation of their specific configuration, i.e. of their RNA, into a DNA copy. Only the latter is then integrated into the genome of the nucleus of the affected cell. Here replication now takes place. Afterwards, and after it has left the nucleus, it is changed back into RNA. This process of 'transferral' (transcription) of RNA into DNA is unusual. The virus contains its own specific enzyme for this purpose, the reverse transcriptase. Only after it starts to work can the reverse flow of information from the cell body into the nucleus take place. Information normally flows from the head to the metabolic system, genetic information from the nucleus to the cell body. In this special case the information flow is reversed from the metabolism to the head, from the cell body to the nucleus. That is why these viruses are usually called retroviruses (Engl.: 'reverse poison').

In all three cases, with the DNA viruses, the RNA viruses and the retroviruses, the replicated virus particles leave the host cell, wrapped in parts of the cell membrane of the latter in some cases, and are now in a position, as mature viruses, to infect other cells.

The *AIDS virus* belongs to the retroviruses, to the RNA viruses. Their RNA genome is significant initially as the provider of information for the metabolism, i.e. the HIV virus has a relationship (tropism) with the perceptual structures of the metabolic sphere. This explains the tendency specifically to affect lymphocytes. But at the same time its character as a retrovirus with the transcription of its RNA into DNA and its insertion into the genome of the host cell indicates the relationship of this virus to the head structure. This explains the neurotropism of this virus and its tendency to affect the cells of the central nervous system. After the HIV virus has replicated in the affected cells, it leaves them. The latter die off in this process, although their death is linked quantitatively to the number of viruses leaving the cell.[70]

If we look at the stages we have dealt with above and place them in the context of our study of the human being, the following picture emerges: throughout life invading structures from the environment are perceived as alien on a microbiological level by the immunological structure of the lymph system and eventually digested after a step-by-step process of immunological recognition and resistance, i.e. they are overcome by the biological self. Throughout the organism the permanent world structures which have been imprinted on the immunological memory (world-representation) interpenetrate the specific individual characteristics of the biological self (self-representation).

In sexual fertilization, an alien structure, the genome of the male spermatozoon, is introduced into the female organism in a process initially comparable with the immune system. Since the ovum does not represent a part of the immunological structure of the (female) biological self, but, on the contrary, is removed from the tissue and, eventually, the supersensory elements of the maternal organism, as part of its maturing processes, immunological recognition does not take place. Thus 'self' and 'alien' do not meet in fertilization, as they do in immunological recognition, but rather 'alien' meets 'alien'. This process does not take place in the sphere governed by the biological self; it is no longer integrated into the latter. It takes place in isolation. In this 'isolation' (R. Steiner [71]) it is simultaneously a process which takes place in the world, a process which can be influenced by cosmic forces. Rudolf Steiner therefore calls fertilization an exposure to cosmic forces. The unification of the male and female genome represents the primal perception, the initial perceptual contact with the material sphere, of the child's supersensory constituent elements which are constructed from these cosmic forces. At the same time the digestive process which we called primal nourishment develops. For the ingestion of the fertilized

70   Cf. Gallo, *loc. cit.*, note 63.
71   Cf. Steiner, *loc. cit.*, note 64.

ovum as the very first material substance to enter the spiritual organism of the child represents the start of material nourishment. Perception and digestion therefore become one in fertilization (see Diagram 10).

Viruses which manage to enter a host and, like the retroviruses, replicate in the genome of the host cell are imitating the fertilization process. But it has been doubly modified:

1. Unlike the genome contained in human spermatozoa, the viral genome contains sub-human information which cannot be completed by human hereditary substance. It uses the vital processes of the nucleus of the host cell merely as a 'stowaway'. Therefore no sexual recognition, no primal perception takes place. Fertilization thus takes place with a 'false seed'.

2. With AIDS, fertilization does not take place in the ovum, but in an immunocyte. These cells are not part of a fixed section of tissue but are mobile and wander through the organism. They have not been 'isolated' — like the sex cells — from the supersensory forces of the biological 'I', but serve the immunological self. That is why they cannot be exposed to the cosmos; detoxification through primal digestion cannot take place.

With AIDS, then, fertilization takes place in an organic and cellular sphere where it was not intended; it has been dislocated, moved to the wrong organ. Furthermore, fertilization does not take place through a human 'poison' which can be detoxified through the cosmic development of a human being. On the contrary, the sub-human poison which enters through this kind of fertilization destroys the human being; the AIDS seed is deadly.

As we noted earlier, all inflammatory processes are displaced digestive processes, all allergic illnesses are 'out of place' perception. With AIDS, on the other hand, we are dealing with displaced fertilization — pathological, fatal fertilization.

CHAPTER SIX

THE DUAL NATURE OF HUMAN BEINGS. AN ESOTERIC EPIDEMIOLOGY WITH REFERENCE TO AIDS

Epidemics: are there 'external' demonic forces in nature?

AIDS — like all epidemics which have affected mankind — is more than just a scientific and medical problem. With epidemics, doctors are dealing not only with individual patients but with a pathogenic entity of a more general kind.[72] Although this can be said of all human illnesses, it is particularly true of epidemics. There are social and psychological problems associated with them which can, under certain circumstances, affect all mankind. Illnesses can be described by the way in which they affect an individual person, showing clearly defined symptoms and a predictable course. But with epidemics, this description must include an understanding of the way the disease spreads through populations, 'among the people' *(epi-demios)*.

The periods preceding modern natural science perceived a particular spirit, a dynamic law, a demonic will in the spread of such epidemics. That is why they referred to the *'genius epidemicus'*.[73] People thought they recognized supernatural

---

72 Rudolf Steiner, *Spiritual Science and Medicine*, Rudolf Steiner Press, London 1948.
73 Jacques Ruffié/Jean-Charles Sournia, *Die Seuchen in der Geschichte der Menschheit*, Stuttgart 1987.

motives behind this 'genius' — divine retribution, predestined fate, the forces of history. The nineteenth century introduced a wealth of discoveries and scientific knowledge into this world of vague assumptions or heroic convictions, which developed into the basis for the modern study of infectious diseases. Just as microscopic observation[74] opened up a whole new world of invisible structures in the study of the human being, so a new invisible realm of nature with all its subdivisions and differentiation was uncovered outside the human being. It could be demonstrated that the influence, the invasion of such micro-organisms — so-called infectious germs — plays a significant role in infectious epidemics.

For medical science the so-called pathogens became the natural cause for a great number of illnesses, the infectious diseases.[75] Medicine at the start of this century, intoxicated with its belief in progress, thought it had solved — at least theoretically — the problem of epidemics. The therapeutic concept could be set out scientifically and microbiologically: *'Therapia magna sterilisans'*. The more it became possible — people thought — to kill off the pathogens around and within human beings, to create a 'sterile' environment in this sense, the more the 'final victory' over the epidemics affecting mankind was within reach. In the first instance, this concept was applicable only to one group of pathogens, the bacteria. Viruses, in contrast, could not be conquered by such sterilizing treatment. The measure which was developed at more or less the same time to deal with them was the present-day prophylaxis of immunization, preventative vaccination. It seemed that the right path had been found which put the eradication of all epidemics from mankind within sight and reach. The appearance of AIDS has dimmed such hopes again. The peculiar characteristics of the HIV virus do not permit the rapid control of the epidemic. Effective immunizing vaccines are not in sight. The situation demands a rethink about the nature of epidemics. How can we understand that the AIDS virus, a 'false seed' in the 'wrong place', leads to

---

74 See Chapter One.
75 Ernst Wiesmann et al, *Medizinische Mikrobiologie*, Stuttgart/New York 1986.

fatal fertilization? What is the background to the appearance of this venereal disease, this fatal epidemic.

These questions are of concern to many people, and when Robert Gallo — one of the foremost AIDS researchers — poses the question at the end of his scientific report on AIDS:[76] 'Is there a moral to be drawn from this terrible business?', the answer pursues a specific direction: 'Yes. One of the frequently quoted glorious achievements of science in the last two decades has been the eradication of infectious diseases — at least in the rich, industrialized nations. The appearance of retroviruses, which are capable of causing an extraordinarily complex and devastating illness, has exposed this supposed victory as the deceptive overestimation of its capabilities. Nature never really allows itself to be defeated; the human retroviruses and their complicated interaction with human cells are only one example of that. Perhaps "victory" is indeed the wrong term to describe our relationship with nature: after all, it does more than surround us; in the final instance we are also part of it.'

It is true, of course, that human beings are part of nature, but they are also spiritual entities. And this dual nature of the human being, which both embeds him in nature and raises him above it, has to be taken into consideration when we attempt to answer questions about illness, disease and epidemics. Otherwise, these kinds of questions will remain unanswered. Medicine as a natural science cannot on its own solve the epidemiological riddles; a supersensory, an 'esoteric epidemiology' also needs to be developed. Human existence comprises both natural and historical processes. It is an illusion to describe these two levels as occurring in parallel but in absolute separation from one another, to understand them as two separate things. It is the purpose of a comprehensive anthroposophical anthropology to investigate and comprehend the laws which connect them. This includes an epidemiology based on the science of the spirit, an esoteric epidemiology. We will develop the outline of such an epidemiology below, particularly in respect of the AIDS epidemic.

Adolf Portmann has drawn attention to the questions with

---

76 Robert Gallo, 'Das AIDS-Virus', in: *Spektrum der Wissenschaft*, vol.3/1987.

which we are concerned here.[77] He describes one of the most dangerous viral illnesses to affect human beings and some animals: rabies. The virus, which enters the organism through a bite from a rabid animal or person, is very specific in the way it spreads through the organism. The symptoms, which primarily affect the central nervous system, are heightened aggressiveness, an irresistible frenzy to bite, the urge to roam and an extraordinary aversion to water. In addition, there are muscle spasms of the throat which prevent swallowing. This strange combination of very different symptoms and pathological forms of behaviour turns out to be the result of the selective action of the rabies virus in the brain. Its coherence becomes clear when we look at the consequences.

The virus, which is particularly present in the saliva of the infected person or animal, is spread most effectively through the combination of all the actions described above. For the sick person's aggressive frenzy to bite guarantees the introduction of saliva, and thus the virus, into the tissue of new victims; the extraordinary drive of the patient to roam ensures that it becomes widely spread; the hydrophobia and muscle spasms in the throat prevent the virus from being made harmless through swallowing. The whole nervous organism of the patient has been reprogrammed to spread and thus multiply the virus; it serves — to use Portmann's expression — an 'heteronomous purpose'. This astonishing process causes Portmann to remark that 'in the case of rabies, the simplest form akin to living structures that we know forces into its service the highest form of life on earth, the human being, in a way which cannot but be described as demonic.' The peculiar 'wisdom' of the virus, which forces the highly complex functions of the human nervous system, and thereby the whole human being, into its service is described by Portmann, following E. Neumann, as 'external knowledge'. A logic, a coherence of action, is meant by this term, which is evident throughout nature independent of and outside human consciousness.

It is not, of course, manifest only in viruses and their

---

77 Adolf Portmann, *Biologie und Geist*, Frankfurt/Main 1973, Chapter Seven.

'behaviour'. Their egotistical 'intelligence' only comes as such a surprise because it is unexpected in view of the exceptionally small size and the relative primitiveness of their structure. The 'demonic' nature of their action lies in this striking discrepancy between formal primitiveness on the one hand and extreme functional complexity on the other. Can we redefine the concept of an 'external' intelligence, of demonic forces in nature, independent of past traditions of thought, in a way which enables us to make sense of phenomena such as rabies or, specifically, AIDS?

Macro-forms in the realms of nature

The whole of visible nature can be seen as a graded structure comprising four realms of nature, although the boundaries and transition points between them may be blurred. The mineral realm, a world of inorganic, dead matter, forms the basis on which a hierarchy of three other living realms is built: plants, animals and human beings. Without going into a detailed consideration of the wealth of phenomena which can justify such a division, we will concentrate here on some characteristics which are of significance in the present context.[78]

Diagram 12

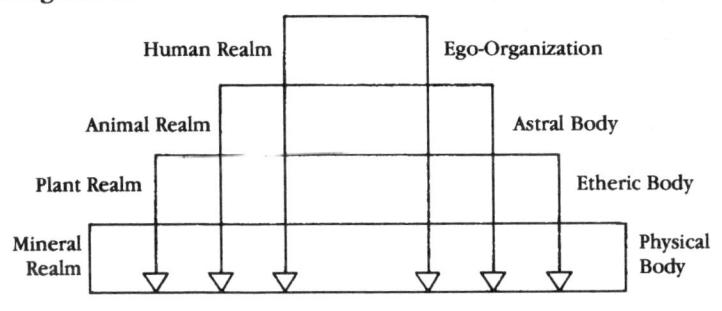

```
              Human Realm            Ego-Organization
         Animal Realm                  Astral Body
    Plant Realm                            Etheric Body
Mineral                                        Physical
Realm                                          Body
```

[78] Rudolf Steiner and Ita Wegman, *Fundamentals of Therapy*; Hermann Poppelbaum, *Mensch und Tier*, Dornach 1975; Otto Julius Hartmann, *Die Gestaltstufen der Naturreiche und das Problem der Zeit*, Halle/Saale 1945; Friedrich A. Kipp, *Die Evolution des Menschen im Hinblick auf seine lange Jugendzeit*, Stuttgart 1980; Wolfgang Schad, *Säugetier und Mensch*, Stuttgart 1971; cf. also Chapter Two.

As we have shown above, there is a radical qualitative leap as we progress from the lower to the higher realms of nature. This is due to the action at each level of a higher supersensory structure which affects and penetrates the lower structures. The leap from the mineral to the plant realm rests on the intervention of the etheric body, the structure which organizes the life forces. It penetrates the physical body, i.e. the structure which organizes the processes of mineral substances. On the animal level these two structures are penetrated by the astral body, i.e. the structure which comprises the internal feelings, and on the human level this is supplemented by the ego-organization of the 'I'. At each of these stages the highest of the elements we have described is dominant. We are not therefore dealing with a progression in which one realm of nature is added to the next, but with the penetration of the lower organizational level by a higher organizational principle, in which the latter is dominant.

This dominance is expressed in two ways: in the transformation of matter and in the transformation of form. Each individual form in the four realms of nature passes through a more or less invisible 'germ stage' in its development. The macro-form only appears as the final stage of the formative principle which is active in the transformation of matter. This applies, as we know, to the living plant, animal and human worlds; but it is also true of the mineral world. A *crystal*, for example, also passes through a kind of germinal stage before growing to a visible dimension. In contrast to living forms, this crystal growth is purely spatial and quantitative. The crystal form, which is already present in the 'germ', merely undergoes identical enlargement without any change in shape. The *plant* also develops from a germ — but into a living form. This living form unfolds — like the crystal — into space, but also into the dimension of time through steady change, in accordance with certain laws (metamorphosis). The temporal form of the plant is characterized by the cyclical recurrence of the same formal stages throughout the year (vegetation cycle). If the plant's life structure penetrates inorganic matter the latter is removed from the mineral state and raised to the level of living substance. At the same time the etheric structure takes on visible form in the shape of the plant. Form at the level of mineral substance is profoundly changed through the intervention of the etheric structure: crystal shape and plant shape in their impressive difference are the visible expression of the qualitative leap from the mineral to the plant realm.

Animals, too, pass through an invisible germ stage in their development. They also grow into space and change in the course of time. But they receive their specific animal expression and are organized internally by the presence of a soul. An inner world which is orientated towards the surrounding environment, into which it is firmly integrated, characterizes the living form of the animal as an expression of soul. The plant lives typically in the cycle comprising the formal metamorphosis of the vegetation cycle; similarly, animal existence is determined typically by the soul element inhabiting a body. But this habitation is not static; there is a continuous interchange between internal existence and external orientation. Like animals, *human beings* also pass through a germ stage to produce their visible form. The human form can be understood on the basis of the animal one if we recognize that not only a soul structure has been created and inhabits it, but that the incarnation of a central being has occurred. The human 'I' — unlike the astral structure of the animal — is not firmly harnessed into the relationship between internal world and environment, but develops an internal autonomy. This becomes effective on a functional level in the autonomy of the temperature-regulating mechanism, and also in the immune system. Finally, it is expressed visibly in upright posture and other manifestations.

It is the individual constituent elements of each specimen of the plant or animal or human realm which achieve final visibility in the macroscopic form of a plant, an animal or a human being. Thus each plant is an expression of that particular specimen's underlying etheric body, each animal, each human being of their underlying astral body and 'I' respectively. But with minerals the only thing which becomes visible is the principle which organizes the physical structure. The clearest example of this is the crystal shape.

However, it is the phenomena at the boundaries between the

realms of nature which are of particular interest. There it becomes evident that the next higher element exercises some influence on the lower realm before this is expressed in the relevant shape. Thus, for example, we find a typical expression of ego organization — the independent temperature-regulating mechanism — in the higher vertebrates (warm-blooded animals) although these animals do not possess an independent 'I'. If they did, this qualitative leap would be expressed in the change of form from animal to human being. A similar effect — here of the astral nature of the animals — can be found in the plant world. The essential animal nature overlaps with the sphere of flowering plants in the blossom, so that the latter is functionally affected from the outside without thereby transforming the plant as a whole into an animal. The plant does not possess an astral *body*; the surrounding astrality merely affects it in the blossom. We therefore have to make a distinction when we observe the realms of nature between the elements which form part of the constitution of a given specimen and the effects of the next higher element which is not part of that constitution. The functional quality which appears in the animal realm as a body-building influence (astral body) is effective in the environment of the plant organism in the plant realm and affects it as an environmental influence.

There are many examples of such anticipation of a higher functional principle on the preceding level in the realms of nature, but they cannot be enumerated here. Such an effect can also be described — as Portmann says — as 'external'. An incorporated constituent element works 'internally', i.e. from the inside and its actions extend to the transformation of the form. External action touches the structure from the outside and therefore only intervenes on a functional level. In contrast to the incarnated, embodied element, the external action is not organized individually; it is not a 'body'. On the contrary, it is part of the environment of the plant, the animal or the human being; it is supra-individual and acts on the group as a whole. It does not determine the form of the specimen but merely its behaviour, i.e. its relationship with the external environment. For example, each individual specimen in the animal world

Diagram 13

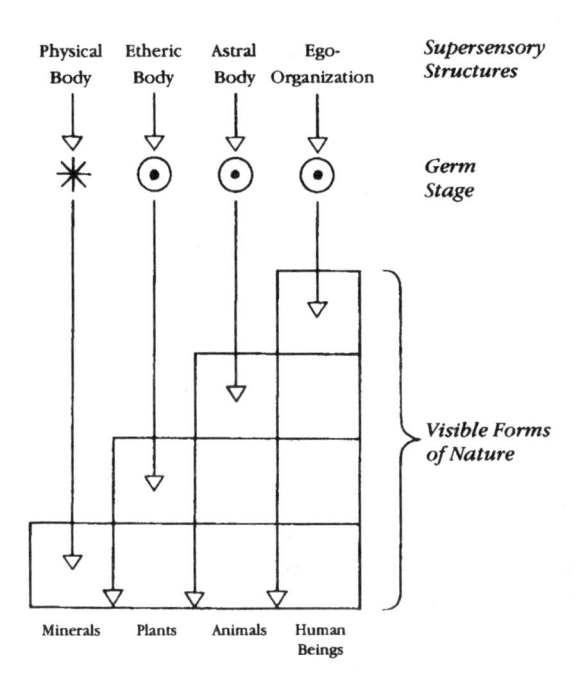

	Physical Body	Etheric Body	Astral Body	Ego-Organization	*Supersensory Structures*

Germ Stage

Visible Forms of Nature

Minerals Plants Animals Human Beings

incorporates an astral body. In contrast, the 'I' principle affects the whole group supra-individually from the outside. It can therefore be described as a spiritual characteristic of the group; it is the 'I' of each animal species.

This unconscious spiritual characteristic, which is revealed in the instinctive modes of animal behaviour uncovered by behavioural research, is nothing other than the external wisdom which is specifically present in the environment. It is the spiritual characteristic of the 'I' on a level appropriate to the animal stage, the group-spirit of the animals.

One of the primary aims of scientific research which has been expanded by Anthroposophy is to work out as clearly as possible

Diagram 14

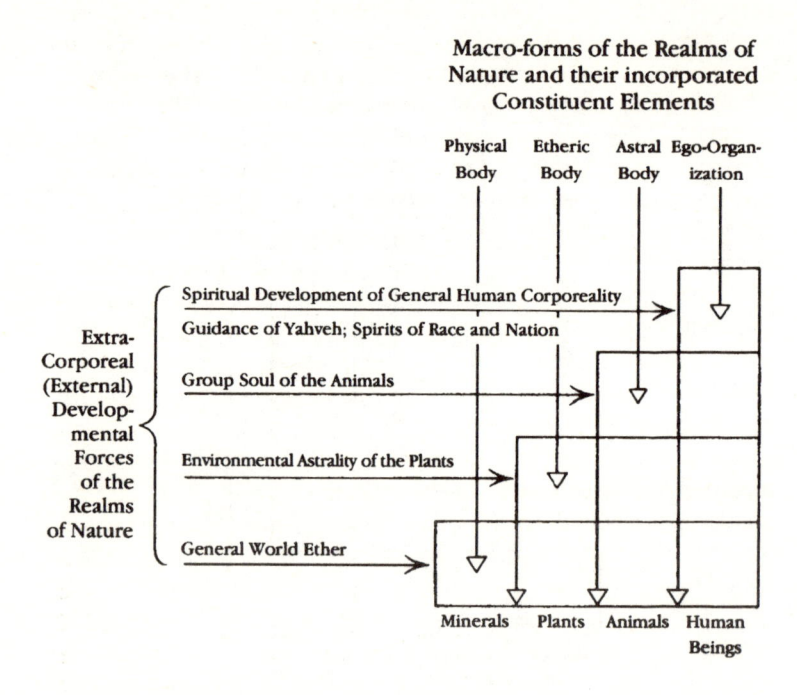

Macro-forms of the Realms of Nature and their incorporated Constituent Elements

```
                                    Physical   Etheric   Astral   Ego-Organ-
                                      Body      Body     Body     ization
```

Extra-Corporeal (External) Developmental Forces of the Realms of Nature	Spiritual Development of General Human Corporeality
	Guidance of Yahveh; Spirits of Race and Nation
	Group Soul of the Animals
	Environmental Astrality of the Plants
	General World Ether

Minerals Plants Animals Human Beings

the differences between incarnated formative and life processes and spiritual actions at work outside the body. Here we can merely give an outline of the principle behind this structure of the realms of nature.

The counter-world of the micro-structures

The structures of the micro-world do not become visible forms. They remain at the germ stage, a stage which each single specimen of the macro-forms of the realms of nature merely passes through (see Diagram 14). The micro-organisms, also called *protista*, therefore do not develop macro-forms which would be suitable for the incarnation of spiritual elements. Their vital functions are largely under the external control of formative forces outside the body; they are really nothing other than the material expression of this external vital activity. Rudolf Steiner also describes these micro-organisms as 'the life process in general' or the 'life of the world in general'.[79]

This description is particularly justified if we take account here of the results of the basic methodological investigation which we described in Chapter One. In contrast to the macro-forms of the living world, the micro-organisms whose existence was uncovered by experimental microscopy require a 'complementary knowledge'. The individual cell, the individual bacterium, etc., has to be returned to the context from which it was isolated through the use of the microscope. In this sense the individual micro-organism is devoid of reality until it is cognitively lodged back in its context of external forces, which Rudolf Steiner, as we said, calls the life process in general, thereby returning the micro-organism to its specific reality. When we are dealing with the macro-forms which exist in the realms of nature, we can, by means of our objective knowledge, describe the individual plant, the individual animal, in every detail within the context of its type as manifest in visible form. The supersensory structure of the body has become visible, it is incarnated. The external, functional context in which the micro-organisms are embedded can only be grasped by supersensory observation which is independent of perception because the functional context does not become visible as 'body'.

As regards a classification of the micro-structures, the question of their connection with the realms of nature — the minerals, plants, animals and human beings — arises over and above any attempt at a biological classification. While the realms of nature develop macro-forms, the micro-organisms remain, as we saw, at the germ stage. But they develop certain physiological characteristics within this germ stage which allows us to classify them in accordance with the realms of nature.

The *protista* can be classified into: protozoa (unicellular

---

[79] Rudolf Steiner, *Schicksalszeichen auf dem Entwicklungswege der Anthroposophischen Gesellschaft*, Dornach 1943, address of 13 August 1914.

organisms), bacteria and viruses. Whereas protozoa represent unicellular organisms which contain a nucleus (eukaryots), the classical cell is polarized one-sidedly into its component parts in the bacteria and viruses: bacteria largely consist of cytoplasm which has fragments of nucleus embedded in it (prokaryots). In contrast, viruses consist of nuclei which have fragments of protoplasm attached. [80] An investigation of the relationship between protozoa, bacteria and viruses and the realms of nature provides us with the following observations:

Bacteria are in the purest sense the material expression of the life process in general. Their importance for the life processes as a whole on earth is immeasurably great. They inhabit the oceans and the earth's surface, as well as the atmosphere. Their formless metabolism is exceedingly diverse and affects the existence of plants, animals and human beings, as well as the mineral and geological transformation of matter. For example, soil bacteria release 92×10^9 tonnes of CO_2 gas annually from the quantities of gas (129×10^9 tonnes annually) fixed assimilatively by the plant world. [80] The activity of the plant world thus directly counteracts the activity of the bacteria. Together they form the central element in the 'carbon cycle' which passes through the soil, the hydrosphere and the atmosphere. The predominance of living metabolic activity therefore classifies bacteria on the level of the plant world, although as an anti-world.

The *protozoa* participate in this formless general world metabolism. Nevertheless, they display a tendency, in contrast to the bacteria, to include large quantities of mineral substance in their metabolic activity and to deposit it in their micro-structure. This explains how the great sections of sedimentary rock in the mountains and on the ocean floor are made up of the dead bodies of mineral metabolizing protozoa. This shows a clear link between protozoa and the mineral realm, but nevertheless as an anti-realm.

The *viruses*, which have been characterized as freely roaming genes, are removed from the sphere of the living metabolism. They themselves do not develop any metabolic activity, which means that they are not truly living beings. Their multiplication

---

80 Hans G. Schlegel, *Allgemeine Mikrobiologie*, Stuttgart/New York 1985.

AIDS — THE DEADLY SEED

Diagram 15

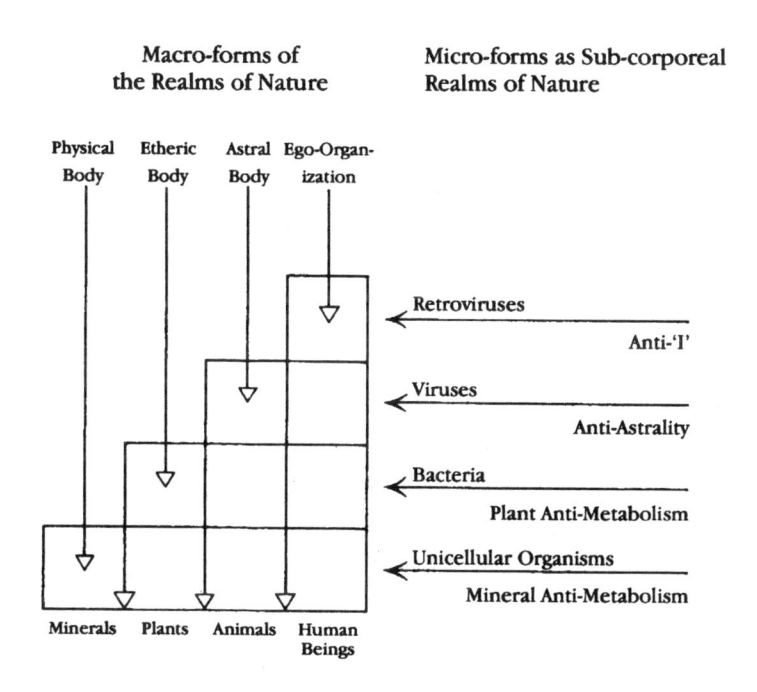

Macro-forms of   Micro-forms as Sub-corporeal
the Realms of Nature   Realms of Nature

| Physical | Etheric | Astral | Ego-Organ- |
| Body | Body | Body | ization |

← Retroviruses
    Anti-'I'

← Viruses
    Anti-Astrality

← Bacteria
    Plant Anti-Metabolism

← Unicellular Organisms
    Mineral Anti-Metabolism

Minerals Plants Animals Human Beings

takes place merely parasitically on the basis of an already existing foreign life-process. Thus viruses can multiply in the cell bodies of prokaryots (bacteria) and eukaryots (uni- and multicellular organisms). Since their substance accords to nuclear substance, they perform the function of RNA when they are inoculated into a cell, i.e. they determine the specific direction of the metabolic activity of the cell in accordance with a 'heteronomous purpose'. The reprogramming of the cell metabolism by the viral genome serves to replicate the virus, to spread its influence. And this influence has a specifically toxic character which has a paralysing, deadening effect on the life of the affected organism. This very specific destructive effect of a micro-toxin which has no life of its own, places the viruses on a par with the astrality of the animal world. For the astral body which we find in animals assumes the characteristics of a poison towards the generative activity of the life body. The pure vitality which characterizes plants is hemmed in in animals and broken down — and in being broken down it is given a specific direction — through the astral body. The generalized life-process is orientated in a specific direction through the incumbent astral body. The nature of viruses can be equated with these actions of animal astrality. But there is a decisive difference. The organized astral body of the animal determines the 'biological self' of the animal, indeed, it is identical with the latter. With a virus, however, an alien, external astrality invades the affected organism. Unicellular organisms correspond in a certain sense to the mineral realm and bacteria to the plant realm; similarly the viruses correspond to the animal realm, forming an astral anti-realm.

Bearing in mind our earlier description of the particular, toxic effects of *retroviruses*, particularly the HIV virus, certain conclusions become inevitable. The AIDS virus, as we noted earlier, affects not only specific organs, as tends to happen with the various viral tropisms, but the structure of the 'I' in one of its most intensive forms, the lymphatic and blood systems. For the activity of the biological self is concentrated in the latter in the form of immunological resistance. Whereas viruses are generally the carriers of unformed environmental astrality and its toxic action, a kind of unformed ego spirituality of the environment, which can also be described as an anti-'I', appears to activate its microinstrument in the retroviruses.

In conclusion, the world of the micro-organisms can be seen as a *counter-world* to the formed world of the realms of nature. The external, formless forces in which the micro-organisms are embedded have a dissolving effect on the mineral world (protozoa), a liberating effect on the large quantity of compounds fixed by the plant world (bacteria), and a toxic effect on the inner world of animals and human beings (viruses). This shows unicellular organisms, bacteria and viruses to be the invisible, material agents of supersensory effects whose origin requires investigation by the science of the spirit.

AIDS — THE DEADLY SEED

Diagram 16

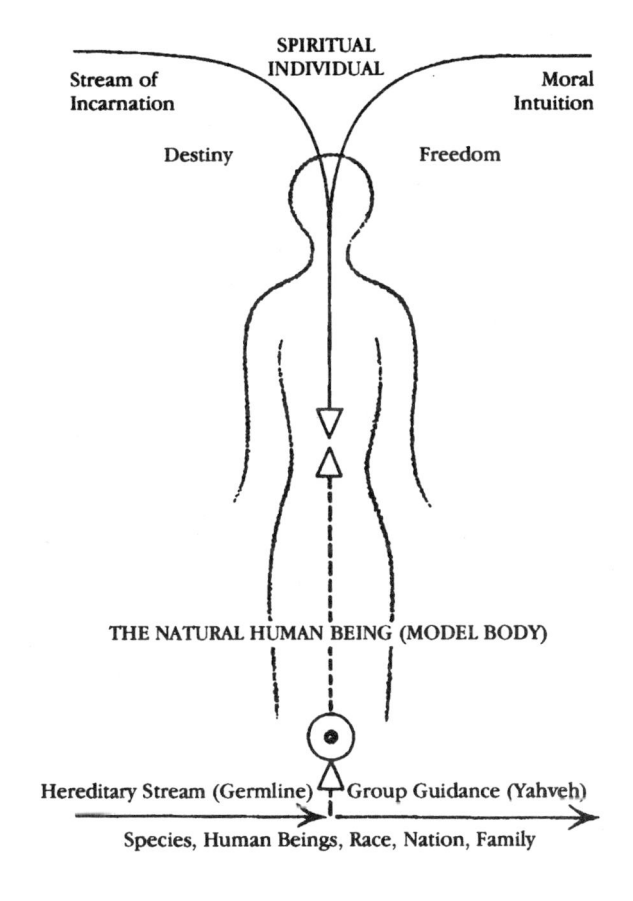

SPIRITUAL INDIVIDUAL

Stream of Incarnation — Moral Intuition

Destiny — Freedom

THE NATURAL HUMAN BEING (MODEL BODY)

Hereditary Stream (Germline) — Group Guidance (Yahveh)

Species, Human Beings, Race, Nation, Family

The human being — a dual being

The position of human beings in nature is a curiously double one. Conception and heredity make him part of the species *man*. Every single human being is a representative of this species and its subdivisions. He is a specimen of a human being, his race, his people, his family. Incarnation and individual destiny (karma) make him an individual, and as an individual 'each person is a species unto himself '.[81]

At incarnation, i.e. during the process in which the individual as a spiritual being begins to inhabit an inherited body, a structure is made available which itself contains all the constitutional forces of the human being. The inherited body is not a sub-human structure but is permeated by forces which have been integrated from the four stages which comprise the realms of nature. Anthroposophy also refers to this four-stage human body as the *model body*. Incarnation, starting with conception, consists of the gradual penetration of the model body by the individual 'I', astral body and etheric body, as well as the individually formed spiritual seed of the physical body.[82]

The model body is composed of an inherited physical body, etheric body, astral body and an inherited ego-organization. Together they form the human being, but this model human being is subject to certain outside guidance on a soul-spiritual level; as a member of the human species he is guided by the group instincts of his race, people and family. The science of the spirit shows how the leading spiritual guiding power of this hereditary generic human being was active from primal times in guiding hereditary man along the paths intended by original creation.[82]

The parameters which determine human nature through racial and national characteristics are integrated as such under this general leading spiritual power. But this spiritual power later appeared historically as the guide of a particular ('chosen') people, the Jews. From this we can also call this spiritual being

---

81 Rudolf Steiner, *Theosophy*, Chapter Two.
82 Rudolf Steiner, *Occult Science*, Chapter 'Man and the Evolution of the World'.

Yahveh or Jehovah. In this respect Yahveh is the god of human creation through reproduction and heredity. He is — as is shown by the Jewish understanding of God — the creator of the human 'I' as an element of the species, as an unconscious, spiritual group entity through the hereditary stream, that is, through the model body. According to the biblical text, which is based on spiritual insight, Yahveh-Elohim is the spiritual being who forms man as the model human being on earth ('of the dust of the ground'), introduces the duality of the sexes and thus ensures sexual reproduction.

At conception a human individual is incarnated into this visible bodily vehicle, of which millions of specimens exist, and individualizes the general model body through the course of its life. The transformation of the model body is both a process of physiological development and a significant biographical event. There are numerous physical and mental aspects to the penetration of the model body by the individual, in the sense of the dual nature of the human being. One particular aspect, to be dealt with separately here, is sexual maturity. When sexual maturity is reached in the third seven-year period, the asexual human individual incarnates into a specific male or female model body. To put it another way, the individual human being becomes immersed in the bodily sphere of sexuality, formed and governed by Yahveh.

In the course of human history the importance of the spiritual individual has increased in relation to the generalized human body. In contrast, the determinant racial and national characteristics have increasingly lost their previously dominant function in the course of the millennia of human history. The historical process of the liberation of the individual can also be described as a liberation from the dominance of racial, national and general human forces of heredity. Historically, the human spiritual individual has increasingly been able to assert himself. Accordingly the contribution to human civilization as a whole of the forces which formed the races and determined national and familial characteristics has undergone a clear, degenerative change, particularly in recent times.

The problems facing human civilization today can thus be

understood by observing, among other things, the degenerating formative forces of race and nation and, indeed, of the model body in general on the one hand, while bearing in mind the weakness and frailness of the spiritual individual on the other. Although the latter has been able to assert the principle of individual self-determination against all the forces of race and heredity in its grand march of liberation well into the twentieth century, it has so far developed only a small measure of the spiritual strength required to fill creatively the space thus conquered and to develop an independent soul-spiritual culture which takes account of the individual.

Many symptoms indicate that the incarnation of the soul-spiritual individual into the model body has been less deep since the start of the twentieth century than in earlier times. Powerful personalities have tended to benefit from this 'loosening'; their creative spirit is less encumbered and impeded by the degenerative nature of the model body. This is not the case with frailer individuals; the weakening of group guidance through the body and its supra-individual laws makes this frailty more apparent than with an 'I' which is deeply incarnated.

A specific symptom of this historical process is evident in human sexuality with the increase in *homophilia*. The souls of individuals who, as they reach sexual maturity, fail to incarnate into the body far enough to reach the clearly defined level of male or female physical characteristics prepared by the forces of Yahveh, remain at the stage of sexual indeterminacy. On a soul and physical level they fail to advance to the fully developed polarity of the sexes. This state of indeterminacy forms the basis for homosexual behaviour.

There are therefore, as we can see, a number of aspects to the looser *incarnation* which is necessary — and will become ever more necessary for the future of mankind — for the *development of the free spiritual individual*. While the guidance of and determination through the supra-individual spiritual forces of the physically-bound civilizations is reduced, the free individual is not yet strong enough to find his own orientation and support himself by his own strength in the indeterminate, intermediate realm which he inhabits above the realm of nature. That was not so in ancient cultures such as the Hebraic. Unlike the Greeks, for example, the ancient Jews, who, in particular, were guided by the spiritual being, Yahveh, punished homophilia with death.[83] A spiritual guiding force whose task in human development lay wholly in the sphere of sexual reproduction and heredity could not tolerate sexual indeterminacy. That can also lead us to an understanding of the general strictness of Jewish culture. With the Greeks there was a natural loosening in the extent of incarnation. That explains the markedly different disposition which made possible the artistic colourfulness and multiplicity of Greek culture.

The growing disconnection between body and soul is increasingly tolerated today and we may postulate that it is only a symptomatic expression of a development which will culminate in the cessation of human physical reproduction on earth through interaction between the two sexes.[84]

The actions, the behaviour of the *model human being* are subject to supra-individual guidance: the 'law' endowed by Yahveh. This guidance works through a form of spiritual heredity which is tied to race and nation, that is, to traditions passed on through the circumstances of birth.

By comparison, human *individuality* is the bearer of individual morality. And this individual morality develops through the laws of destiny (karma) in the same way as the human being in the state of nature is both created and guided by the laws of heredity.[82] The concept of individual morality is so easily misunderstood today that a clarification of the term seems advisable. It does not mean the individual adherence to ideological or social moral prescriptions. These — however justified — are still group characteristics. Individual morality develops on the basis of the independent intuition of each human being and is not bound by any traditions.[85] In this sense the term means nothing other than the individual capacity for autonomous action. It is creative and

---

83 Information from Dr Benyamin Z. Barsai, Bremen, through Dr Peter Schily, Bochum, Germany.
84 Rudolf Steiner, *Building Stones for an Understanding of the Mystery of Golgotha*, Rudolf Steiner Press, London 1972, lectures of 10 and 12 April 1917.
85 Rudolf Steiner, *The Philosophy of Freedom*, Chapter Nineteen.

only binding on the person of whom it is an expression. Something new enters the world with every person who uses this source as the basis of their action. In this sense morality and freedom are identical. Yet the degree of moral intuition is dependent on the degree of karmic experience a person has gathered through destiny. Thus the force of destiny and individual freedom also meet at the point of moral intuition.

The transformation of the model human being through the individual human being and his morality, starts at the point of incarnation and continues throughout life. Here we may note a particular rhythm: the daily action of waking up and falling asleep. Waking up in the morning is a daily mini-incarnation and going to sleep in the evening a mini night-time excarnation. And like the contrast between incarnation at waking and excarnation with sleep, the major incarnation at conception and birth contrasts with the great excarnation at death. During the day the influence of the human individuality predominates in the body and makes its mark in accordance with the constitution of its moral consciousness, while during sleep at night those forces predominate which come as external influences from the sphere of the general spiritual nature of humanity which regenerates the body. They renew the body 'in the image of God' to give it the form in which it was once created in his image.

On the origin of demons of illness

We discussed earlier the relationship between the realms of nature, and it became evident that our understanding of nature as matter requires the underlying life forms and forces to become accessible to the senses. As the anatomical structure of an entity becomes simpler and physically approaches the germ stage (or, as with micro-structures, the more it remains at the germ stage), so the research into these stages and structures increasingly requires a supersensory supplement, a complementary knowledge. In order to understand micro-organisms, we therefore need to make greater reference to the anthroposophical science of the spirit. When we think about the results of spiritual scientific research there is one basic requirement, because these results relate to purely spiritual processes and entities. Ordinary thinking, which is nearly always guided by the processes and objects of the sensory world, has to be retrained to become equally practised in handling the purely supersensory content which is provided by spiritual research. This can only happen if scientists, with their cognitive experience, pass through the phase of pure thinking and thereby cross the threshold of sense-bound thought. We outlined such cognitive threshold experiences in Chapter One. Nevertheless, we must draw attention to the methodological steps which lead to complementary knowledge.[86]

One of the most important concepts used by the science of the spirit to describe the underlying processes of nature is *separation*.[87] This refers to a process which can be explained with an example from visible nature. Embryologists have discovered many such processes of separation in human and animal development. The complete development of the nervous system, for example, takes place by separation from the outer germ layer (ectoderm); the same applies to the development of the thyroid gland, the parathyroid gland and the thymus, which all divided from the inner germ layer. The adrenal medulla, too, is an indirect separation of formative substance which previously separated at the same time as the nervous system. The common factor in all these separations is that something subordinate, specific, is differentiated from something more general and comprehensive. The thyroid gland is no longer the whole human being, it is no longer even the whole of the alimentary and metabolic tract, as is the inner germ layer (endoderm) and its associated organs. But it performs a differentiated function in the metabolic system as a whole. Observation of lower animals shows that although they possess a metabolism which indeed shows functional differentiation, it is not differentiated into a number of discrete individual organs. Such organs, then, bring the specific functions which the animal develops in itself, or in

---

[86] See notes 81 and 82; also *Knowledge of the Higher Worlds. How is it achieved?*.
[87] Rudolf Steiner, *The Spiritual Beings in the Heavenly Bodies and in the Kingdoms of Nature*, Anthroposophic Press, New York 1981.

relation to its environment, down to the physical level where they are given bodily-spatial form.

Similar separations occur in the supersensory sphere which complements visible nature, but on an invisible spiritual level. The all-embracing creative spiritual powers of the world separate from themselves dynamic sub-entities for the differentiated individual elements produced by nature, in the same way as the organism as a whole in our example separates specific substructures internally.[88] Supersensory nature therefore appears to spiritual researchers as a hierarchical structure of beings who are situated at various levels, from the highest heights of all-embracing creativity to the simplest individual processes in nature. We cannot here go into the details of such a conception of nature. What is important in our context is the general concept of separation. We will merely pose the question as to whether human beings on a supersensory level help to bring about such separations and of what the latter might consist. We will choose two particular types of separation from the wealth of material provided by Rudolf Steiner, because they are of decisive importance for the creation of 'demons of illness' and thus for an 'esoteric epidemiology'.

1. As we have seen, the individual, the inner moral human being is at work each day in the model human being. He impregnates the instrument of incarnation which nature puts comprehensively at his disposal with the abilities and inabilities which he has — karmically — acquired. When he excarnates in sleep at night he leaves behind the more or less deforming traces of the action of his consciousness. These, for example, may consist of lies, hypocrisy and slander. When the higher spiritual powers, who are engaged during the night in regenerating the organism which has been poisoned and worn out during the day, encounter such deformations, the following happens: 'And the fact that these elements are left in the physical body at night has a special effect. Some of the substance of the beings who enter the body is torn away. As a result, certain parts of the higher beings have to be separated. The result of lying and hypocrisy and

---

88 Cf. Chapter Four

slander during the day is that certain beings arise through separation during the night and as a consequence have a certain affinity with the human physical body. In this way these beings achieve independent existence in the spiritual world which surrounds us ...' Such entities 'will prove to you that it is people's lifestyle which causes beings to arise who do not have a particularly beneficial effect on human beings. For they have qualities of intelligence in certain respects and no moral liability. Their existence consists of creating obstacles for people in their lives; greater obstacles than those we call bacteria. Indeed, something else happens as well. Such beings give rise to important pathogens; for once these phantoms have been created by human beings they find a good basis for existence in bacilli and bacteria, they use them as nourishment, as it were. They would more or less wither in their spiritual existence if this nourishment did not exist. But these bacteria are in turn created by them, in a certain sense.' [89]

In this esoteric context, then, each individual person is the trigger for elemental spiritual entities which arise through separation and which then provide an environment for micro-organisms (bacteria) in which the latter can be embedded as in an external medium of forces. For 'where do the bacilli come from? They are just as much living beings as man. Of those beings too which act as disturbers of human life we must ask: Where do they come from? What has brought them into their present material existence? What were they before they incarnated?' [90]

It would be wrong to conclude from this that the bacteria who are guided in this way will particularly affect the person who participated in their creation in the above sense. That is by no means the case. The significant point here is that an individual person not only affects nature through moral actions exclusively on the territory of his own organism, but that lower nature on an elemental level can be affected via the complicated circuitous route of the processes which occur during sleep; an effect which

---

89 Rudolf Steiner, *Natur- und Geistwesen. Ihr Wirken in unserer sichtbaren Welt* (GA 98), Dornach 1982, lecture of 14 June 1908.
90 Rudolf Steiner, *Foundations of Esotericism*, Rudolf Steiner Press, London 1982, lecture of 3 November 1905.

becomes evident above all in the micro-organisms which act as pathogens on human beings. The latter are even more poisonous (virulent) because of their extraneous orientation.

2. A different form of separation exerts equal esoteric influence on the micro-world: just as the individual human being is excarnated at death, the leading spirit of a nation or race can withdraw from the body of the nation or race. What are the esoteric consequences? 'Let us suppose, for example, that some nation or race is in its decline, is moving towards its downfall. It puts up a resistance. This resistance to its downfall is a spiritual expression of something that lives in the astral body of the nation in question. Were such a decline to concern only that which was to come to an end, then the feeling engendered would have no special effect upon others in the world. Let us assume however that it comes in conflict with another nation, plunging it into fear and anxiety and thus sets up a reaction in this other nation. Then we have a two-fold situation: the nation suffering decline, and what arises out of the confluence of the disturbance of the one people fighting against their own decline, and the fear and alarm of the other people. This is something lasting.'[90] The esoteric consequence of this, once again, is a separation. Rather than the astral nature of a race or nation 'dissolving' in the spiritual world, the clash with another nation leads to a separation; 'spiritual entities' are created. 'Let us take a particular case: the Mongolian onslaughts of the Middle Ages, when the Mongols came into conflict with the Europeans, spreading among them fear and alarm. Such fear and such alarm are then present in the peoples in question. When one looks at these attacking hordes, of which the Mongolians are the last, placing oneself in the mood of all these mediaeval people, one sees how the desperation of the last branches of the Fourth Root Race and the fear and alarm engendered in the Europeans created spiritual forms. If such an onslaught were to be met with courage and love, then the putrefying substances would be dissolved. But fear, hate and alarm conserve such decaying forms and these provide a source of nourishment for beings such as bacilli. Later they incarnate in those material forms suitable for such an incarnation. Thus the decaying substances embedded themselves in the fear and alarm of the European peoples as seeds of decay. These are minute living beings.

In this way arose the mediaeval disease, leprosy. It arose out of the decaying substance of the declining Mongolian peoples. What, then, is the origin of those disturbers of human physical nature? They come from earlier, spiritual causes, from sinfulness. This is Karma as it manifests in national communities. From this you can estimate how the moral life of a nation conditions the external life of the future. It lies in the power of a nation to care for its physical future through a corresponding moral life in the present.' [90]

Such separation is not caused by individual morality but by the morality of the nation or race. Does such a morality exist? If the morality of a people were to be understood as the sum of its parts, it would merely be a quantitative, nominalistic concept. Yet it has become more than apparent, in this century in particular, that the moral strength of an individual is unable to counter the moral weakness of a nation. On the other hand, the moral mission of an individual can sometimes be identical with the mission of this individual's nation in a way which gives the individual moral act an historical dimension. Joan of Arc is one such example. Nevertheless, the connection between national and racial problems and the individual only becomes clear if both these developmental forces working in mankind and in history are seen as strictly separate. It will only be possible to deal in a progressive way with the increasingly apparent problems of race and nationality if we take into account the findings of the science of the spirit which demonstrate that there is a dual aspect to human nature; human beings are part of a group entity determined by environment and heredity on the one hand, and are spiritual individuals on the other. Only this sharp distinction makes it clear that the individual in our age has acquired value and significance independent of the nationality and race into which he has been incarnated.

From additional remarks made elsewhere by Rudolf Steiner about the same process, we can see how little causal connection can be made between the separations arising from the group entity of a race or nation — and the demons of illness which arise as a consequence — and the individual people who are affected by them. He points out that the 'substances of decay' from the Mongol peoples only resulted in leprosy generations later.

Then he continues: 'If we wish to understand this, we must distinguish between the development of a single soul and that of a whole race. The two must not be confused. A human soul can develop in such a way that in one incarnation it embodies itself in a particular race. If in this race it gains certain qualities, it may reimbody itself in a later incarnation in an entirely different one; so that we may find incarnated in Europe at the present day souls which in a previous incarnation were embodied in India, Japan or China. The souls do not by any means remain in the same race, for soul development is quite different from race development.' [91]

As we have seen already, the principle of individuality which outwardly assumes an egotistical form to begin with, becomes increasingly prominent historically. By contrast, national and racial differences become increasingly less important. We can therefore anticipate that the War of All against All 'takes on ever more menacing forms. The things that must come about fulfil themselves with an inner necessity ... It would be senseless to wish to arrest such things. The appropriate and serviceable means to avert the War of All against All was sought by the Theosophical Movement through the spreading of the axiom of brotherhood. For brotherhood dissolves what streams into the world as means of decay, as hate. For as regards race we find ourselves on a downward path. If one were to believe that this downfall could be delayed and contained by hatred, not resolved by love, then naturally the very worst would follow.' [90]

An esoteric epidemiology of AIDS

These words were spoken in 1905. The thoughts expressed both hypothetically and prophetically became reality in the course of the century. The problem of race and the destructive effect of a degenerating nationalistic spirituality have dominated events in this century and still do so. Racial problems exist on almost every continent.

---

91 Rudolf Steiner, *The Spiritual Foundation of Morality*, Steiner Book Centre, Vancouver (no date), lecture of 29 May 1912.

But a conflict between two peoples occurred in the middle of the century which assumed global proportions: *the collision between the Jews and the Germans*. In this context it was simultaneously a racial conflict. If we look at the history of the Jews, we can see a progressive tendency over two millennia for the body of the nation to dissolve and become part of the body of mankind as a whole. This process of assimilation of Jewish culture and the Jews themselves into many nations was developing in a positive fashion in the twentieth century, particularly in the more advanced countries. The ghettoization of the Jews seemed largely overcome. This dis-integration might be described by saying that the special development of the Jews as the chosen people was fully in progress through their assimilation into the whole of mankind. This historical situation was overtaken by the persecution and destruction caused by the German people and their demonic hatred. If the tragedy of the Jews was to hold fast to the spiritual guidance of Yahveh through physical heredity, it was the tragedy of the German people to regress ideologically into the degenerate culture of a nationalistic, indeed, racial spirituality. If — given the history of the twentieth century — we take seriously the words of Rudolf Steiner quoted above, the question immediately arises as to the nature of the 'demons of decay', that is, the spiritual entities which have separated off as a result of this and similar racial conflicts in the twentieth century. AIDS springs to mind!

There can be no doubt that there are many factors in the spiritual genesis of this terrible epidemic which have contributed to its appearance. But its focus can be seen as the conflict between two peoples who have a special relationship to the human 'I'. It was the historical mission of the Jews to give the strongest expression of all peoples to the physical body as the vehicle of the 'I'. The final purpose of this mission was the paramount event of the incarnation of Christ. The history of the German people would be a sorry failure if it were to be judged only in national, political terms. For their disappointing external historical development over the centuries has cloaked an inner historical development, an historical development of the soul, which represents the true mission of this people. This mission consists of developing, in the purest form, an awareness of the 'I' on a soul and spiritual level. The Jewish awareness of the 'I' was based on the physical, hereditary body; similarly the soul-spiritual awareness of human beings, developed particularly by the German people, was based on the warmth body.[92]

In this sense a collision occurred between two peoples with a special commitment to the human self. The demonic hatred shown towards the Jews had to result in decaying substances with particularly toxic effects on the ego-organization. Seen in terms of an esoteric epidemiology, AIDS is the illness through which demons of disease have begun to mount an enormous, unprecedented attack on the human self. Mankind will have to muster all its powers to interpret AIDS as a sign of the times: the *mission of human beings on earth* is at stake, and this mission is a spiritual one, *a mission of the 'I'*.

---

92 Rudolf Steiner, *Erdensterben und Weltenleben* (GA 181), Dornach 1967, lecture of 30 March 1918.

CHAPTER SEVEN

AIDS — INDIVIDUAL DESTINY AND DISEASE

How the patient feels, and medical diagnosis

AIDS, like every illness, possesses a dual perspective: how the patient feels and the medical diagnosis — the patient and the illness. The patient experiences, suffers, the state he is in. The diagnosis is made. If the inner aspect, the state of the patient, were the only thing that existed, it would be easy to believe that we are dealing only with individual patients. The outer aspect, the diagnosis, at first sight recognizes only illnesses.

In his suffering, the patient cannot but ask: 'Why me?' or 'Is that what's in store for me?' [93] The doctor, by contrast, inquires about factors of heredity or the environment, each of which make their contribution to the illness. While nineteenth-century investigation tended on the whole to examine the question of heredity, doctors in the twentieth century have learned to ask about environmental factors, as, for example, Hans Schäfer has done in his book *Plädoyer für eine neue Medizin* (The Case for a New Medicine). [94] Such investigation has also extended the term epidemic to its current usage. While the nineteenth century understood the term as the study of the spread of infectious diseases, today it covers everything connected with an illness resulting from causes beyond the individual patient (*epidemios* = among the people). Thus Schäfer, for example, calls one of the chapters in his book 'Society makes the body ill'.

---

93 'Why me?', series in the news magazine *Der Spiegel*, nos. 34, 35, 36, 37, 38/1987.
94 Hans Schäfer, *Plädoyer für eine neue Medizin*, Munich 1979.

In the previous chapter we tried to show how 'society can make the body ill'. We referred to an esoteric epidemiology, to the spiritual background of catastrophes among nations and races. In natural science, the subject of epidemiology refers to chains and networks of infection in the spread of the disease.

It traces the global spread of the AIDS virus back to areas in central Africa where the disease is endemic. It demonstrates that the links in the chain of this infectious system are both sexual contact and the exchange of blood between people — a key fact for both the scientific and the esoteric epidemiological aspects of the disease. We saw that these perspectives are not mutually exclusive. The nature of micro-organisms [95,96] allows 'spiritual demons of decay' to utilize these entities and guide them 'externally'. Thus an epidemic can spread explosively through the world's population from its latent state in a remote part of the world. The dynamic of the disease does not therefore originate in the infectious material but does make use of it.

Here we will pose the question about individual destiny in relation to AIDS. For the AIDS patient will rightly wonder what connection might exist between himself and the racial conflicts of the twentieth century, in which he, as an individual, may have no involvement by virtue of when and where he lives. These general events probably have as little relevance to him as the scientific report on the origins of the AIDS virus in Central Africa.

But of immediate relevance to the patient, and identical with his own existence, is his particular destiny in relation to the illness. And that is indivisibly connected with him as an individual, as an 'I'. If human beings did not possess a dual nature[96] but were subject only to the forces of nature, the question of their freedom and destiny would be pointless: natural processes would merely be running their course.

Even the clear distinction between sickness and health would be less clear. For both sickness and health would never be more than natural happenings, and nature embraces both regeneration and decline, formation and destruction, evolution and devolution. But with AIDS the conception of the dual nature of

---

95 See Chapter Five.
96 See Chapter Six.

human beings involves asking what this illness means to *this* 'I', irrespective of whether it has acquired the disease as a haemophiliac or a drug abuser, a homosexual or a heterosexual, as a link in one chain of infection or another. Although the latter points are important from an epidemiological point of view, a unique, individual destiny in relation to the illness develops as soon as infection takes place.

AIDS — individual destiny and disease

The core of every human illness can be found in the destiny, in the individuality, of every human being. Destiny is experienced, suffered. How does the AIDS patient experience his fate? [93,97]

Fear is the focus! This fear is nourished from two sources. Fear is caused by the knowledge that one is suffering from an incurable illness irrevocably progressing towards death. But the far-reaching social isolation associated with AIDS also produces fear. Both states of fear — the physical and the social — throw the helpless 'I' back on its own resources. The existential, archetypal relationship of a person to his own body, representing the result of his biographical development from child to adulthood, is profoundly disturbed.

The basic relationship to a loved person, in so far as it is expressed sexually through the body, is also seriously disturbed: the patient has become the carrier of death, instead of the carrier of happiness to the healthy person. There are, of course, other frightening illnesses such as, for example, cancer, whose diagnosis brings with it the threat of death. But AIDS carries the additional threat of social 'solitary confinement' because of the illness.

Other moods and experiences supplement fear as the basic

[97] Karl Heinz Reger/Petra Haimhausen, *AIDS — Die neue Seuche des 20. Jahrhunderts*, Düsseldorf 1985. Hans Halter (ed.), *Todesseuche AIDS*, Hamburg 1985. Frank Rühmann, *AIDS: Eine Krankheit und ihre Folgen*, Frankfurt am Main and New York 1985. August Wilhelm von Eiff/Johannes Gründel, *Von AIDS herausgefordert, Medizinisch-ethische Orientierungen*, Freiburg 1987. Erwin J. Haeberle/Axel Bedürftig, *AIDS — Beratung, Betreuung, Vorbeugung-Anleitung für die Praxis*, Berlin/New York 1987.

temper of the illness: shock at the first diagnosis of the illness, depression, anger, indifference leading to apathy. Deep feelings of guilt can also be accompanied by submission to the inevitable.

On the other hand, a new and previously unknown attentiveness can also set in. One patient described it thus: 'The point is to watch my child develop and to enjoy life for as long as possible. For example, it gives me great pleasure to see how everything has begun to grow, how everything is turning green and blossoming. I live more intensely now because many other things have become less important.' [93] Another patient reported a greater capacity to distinguish between essential and non-essential things in his life.

During the first stage of the illness — with the HIV positive, symptomless patient — the social fear is the most prominent. This is supplemented by the fear of waiting for the appearance of the first symptoms which would bring the illness out into the open. The HIV infected person is not yet sick, but feels the sword of Damocles hanging over him. The illness may break out at any time — but when? He listens in to himself, he watches every commonplace symptom and takes it to be a serious sign. The awareness of the patient is unusually intense and directed towards his own body. And this otherwise familiar body becomes alien through the illness; something 'demonic' has insinuated itself into it.

In the second and third stages,[95] this mood is supplemented by physical difficulties: the patient becomes conscious of weakness, fever, pain, feeling unwell and many different physical complaints. At the full-blown stage all this escalates into a serious experience of ill health which is increasingly felt to be too much to bear.

This whole experience of AIDS, of which we can give only an indication here, provokes a mood in the soul processes of the patient of which he is either intensely aware or otherwise only semi-aware. This mood belongs to the accompanying symptoms of the illness, which are essentially a reflection of something which develops and spreads in the deeply unconscious part of the organism.

But a person's conscious, semi-conscious and organically

unconscious modes of experience, are, in the final analysis, all part of the same thing. They are the consciously reflective and the physically existential modes of existence of the same self. We may thus ask what the individual as a physical entity, as a biological individual, experiences with AIDS. For only half of the course of events which occurs with AIDS is an experience of mental suffering. The other half occurs in the physical organs and takes place in the incarnated constituent elements of the patient. Thus the 'I' of the patient has to fight on two levels, on two fronts: the mental level, at which the patient can speak about his thoughts and experiences, and the organic level which is essentially beyond his awareness.

Let us recall what happens in the organism with AIDS. [95] The physical instrument of the 'I', which it uses in the body to delimit and assert itself against everything alien, everything which is non-'I', is destroyed. The 'I' becomes incapable of distinguishing its own existence from alien matter, to which human beings are continually exposed. The power of immunological recognition of foreign matter which, as we saw, is always linked with self-recognition, is undermined and dwindles away. As a consequence, the self-perception of the 'I' in the organism dwindles to the same extent. The process can be compared to looking in a mirror. A look in the mirror allows us to perceive our physical bodies, but it is necessarily linked with the mirrored environment. If the mirror becomes opaque, self and non-self can no longer be distinguished. Our glance becomes uncertain and indeterminate.

But the immune system does not simply allow the biological distinction between alien matter and the self. We have already demonstrated that, as a subsidiary organization of the blood, it is simultaneously the instrument of the unconscious will which the 'I' uses to resist the invasion of foreign matter and defend the territory of the biological individual. The experience of fading immunological resistance can therefore also be compared with walking in a marsh. The 'I' has lost the supporting ground under its feet, and the body becomes a bottomless swamp with regard to its own actions, with regard to external resistance and self-assertion. With AIDS these processes are of profound importance for the 'I', as they are not only mental experiences but, as we said, belong to the fundamental existential experiences in the unconscious part of the body and its component parts.

The blurring of the frontiers between self and world, the powerlessness of the will, are not apparent to thought processes. They are physically experienced; they are destiny.

About the destiny of being ill

The series of articles in *Der Spiegel* magazine in August/September 1987 about the statements made by AIDS patients from various carrier groups (heterosexuals, homosexuals, haemophiliacs, drug abusers, prostitutes) had as its title the question: 'Why me?' That, indeed, is the key question in every serious illness, and it enquires about the relationship between self and destiny. Is it chance, providence, fate, or commonplace cause and effect? How far am I responsible? How much wrongdoing is contained in my destiny? The lack of an answer to such fundamental questions of human existence, which do not generally receive a great deal of attention, becomes doubly apparent when serious illness occurs, particularly AIDS. The person concerned cannot ignore such questions; his fate poses them inexorably. The way towards an answer requires a delicate approach to the subtle observation of human beings and life. Rudolf Steiner's Anthroposophy can sharpen the senses to look at life, but also to look at the concepts and ideas necessary to understand destiny. We can only give a brief indication here of the spiritual instruments which can lead to an understanding of AIDS. I must also refer to the anthroposophical literature, particularly on the laws of human destiny (karma).[98]

The relationship between world and self is expressed in learning, between self and world in action. Learning provides the self with capacities which change the world through action. But the 'I' cannot transform into action all the experience it gains through interacting with the world.

---

98 Rudolf Steiner, *Theosophy; Occult Science; Luzifer-Gnosis* 1903 — 1908 (GA 34), Dornach 1960; *The Manifestations of Karma*, Rudolf Steiner Press, London 1984.

On the contrary, most experience becomes entangled at various preliminary stages and is retained in a half-digested or completely undigested form. The learning process falters. Only a few experiences become fully assimilated in the innermost part of the 'I'; the others are merely retained in the self's constituent elements as perceptions (physical body), memories (etheric body), subjective pre- and post-conceptions, as well as a wealth of experience-related emotions and feelings (astral body).[99]

All such half-digested experiences, which have failed to be transformed into inner capacities of the 'I', lie in us as 'complexes', as independent 'subordinate structures' of the soul; they are the content of our 'karma', i.e. the preconditions of destiny.

But we do not merely learn, we also act. Through our actions we leave the mark of our innermost abilities, but also of our semi-abilities and inabilities, i.e. our 'complexes', on the world. Whenever a person in a given situation acts on the basis of the full capacities of his 'I', using the power of his individual abilities, his action is in harmony with the world and does not produce any 'complexes', because it fits into the structure of the world. The 'I' is acting on the basis of acquired abilities which lead to a full understanding of the conditions in the world. When people act on the basis of karmically determined complexes, the world is deformed. Such weakness of the 'I' leaves lasting consequences which appear as the force of destiny.

The proper actions of the 'I' take place in a state of freedom. All such free actions are outside destiny, as it were. Thus, something completely new enters the world from the 'I', which is not determined by a previous cause but by an understanding of the given conditions. Such actions are absolutely individual. The decision to take them rests solely with the 'I' that does so.

No one can interfere or participate from the outside in decisions of individual morality.[100] One can only determine afterwards whether the autonomous actions of two 'I's complement one another.[101] If they do so, they were both drawn from free moral intuition. If they were the compulsive result of

---

99 See Chapter Three.
100 See Chapter Six.
101 Rudolf Steiner, *The Philosophy of Freedom*, Chapter Nine.

'complexes' they inevitably clash and exercise a destructive effect on the world.

If free decisions fail to be taken in certain individual biographical situations due to a lack of competence, i.e. through a weakness of the conscious 'I', the complex which arises as a result and its effect on destiny is displaced from the sphere of free decision-making into the area of the body's constituent elements. We move from the sphere of the 'I' into the sphere of the astral body, into the sphere of psychological behaviour. Here we find the whole spectrum of psychological behavioural disorders: psychopathy. Abnormal behaviour, obsessions, feelings of isolation, all types of neurotic disorders can occur. At this stage we have already left the sphere of moral decision making, the sphere of personal free responsibility. We are presented with a pathological mental state which has to be seen essentially as beyond morality. Whereas the 'I' makes its free decisions independently, based completely on its own resources, the above process transforms actions into a social problem because of this primary displacement. Our fellow human being, subject to his psychopathic 'complexes', becomes a social 'obstacle', a permanent 'problem case' and requires our help. This must be educational help but with a medical orientation, that is, curative education.

In this respect the life of such people, their biography, is often an unconscious educational measure which repeatedly aims to awaken the 'I' to independence by causing it to collide with the self-built, self-caused psycho-social obstacles to independence, so that it repeats the failed earlier learning process on a different level.

But destiny-related complexes can be displaced to a second, deeper level. This displacement to the level of the etheric body no longer gives prominence to mental symptoms but to a wealth of physical disorders. These can include feeling unwell, hypochondria, vegetative frailness, and many types of functional debility. For the most part they continue throughout life because — like the psychopathic symptoms — they are constitutional. The patient is not well, but neither is there a concrete organic disorder.

Only with the third displacement does the destiny-related

complex appear in the physical body. Here it causes pain, organic diseases or defects and possibly death. Here, too, the karmic preconditions for infection can gain access to the physical body.

In the second and third displacements it becomes more apparent than in the first displacement that events have been totally removed from the sphere of moral decision making. We are still able to exercise the latter occasionally in a psychopathic condition because the symptoms on this level can oscillate between moral responsibility and subjection to obsessive mental states. But the social aspect of the situation becomes more apparent and more dominant to the same degree as the destiny-related pathological complex in the etheric body, and eventually in the physical body, makes us forget the original moral causes. The illness calls for vigorous care, help and nursing, it demands a therapeutic approach.

The individual's destiny-related complex and its threefold displacement is thus no longer within the free decision-making power of the patient. But that is precisely why free deeds (of love) are required from the community of people within which the patient lives. What started out as a concern of the individual's moral consciousness has become an act of nature and thus demands natural assessment and natural treatment, but within the context of human social coexistence.

The outline we have given here of the illness-related displacement of the individual's original weaknesses and failures is initially true of life in general. 'Problems' are continuously deferred in this sense. The smoker, for example, who perhaps encountered this 'drug' during a personal crisis in his youth, then transfers the problem of that particular phase and it becomes the habit of a lifetime. Finally, in old age he encounters the consequences of transferring the problem on a material level in his body in smoking-related arteriosclerosis.

Such processes, of which we can give only one small example among many, are subject to the laws of what we might call the *localized karma* of someone's life. But in many cases they are insufficient to explain serious, deep-rooted illnesses. At this point Anthroposophy opens up the vista of an individual's repeated lives on earth. Here the displacements take place from one life to the next. Many cases of illness or susceptibility to illness rest on such large-scale and comprehensive displacement from one life on earth to the next.

But these major transformations of karmic complexes will always have superimposed on them the small dislocations which belong to the localized karma of a given life. In the large transformations from life to life the illness has been totally separated from its origin, which at one time had to be seen in moral terms. It has become a factor which simply occurs. With the small dislocations within a single life we can still trace the effects of an illness back to its causes, which may appear as some form of weakness of the 'I', as a cluster of moral decisions.

It is extremely important to realize that all help, care and therapy must be directed exclusively at the illness. The person who wants to help the patient has *nothing* to do with the karmic causes of the latter's illness; that is the concern solely of the sick person. The patient has to be left to deal with the moral and karmic nucleus of his illness because we would otherwise interfere with his freedom as an individual. With regard to the natural and physical consequences of the pathological complex, however, everything humanly possible must be done to prevent, treat or heal the illness.

This twofold aspect of illness, then, 'externally' presents a natural side which lies within the province of the social interaction between human beings; but 'internally' we must ask what 'karmic benefit' the sick person can draw from the illness for his 'I', for his spiritual development. The karmic benefit which the patient can accrue at every stage of the displacements described above is, in the last instance, the deeper, the real meaning of illness as such. For this benefit develops if the 'I' is existentially shaken awake through its encounter with foreign karmic complexes which it experiences physically and in the soul.

The 'I', which has to go through experiences of isolation, failure to be understood, physical weakness, helplessness, pain and all the other illness-related experiences, is thereby engaged in a learning process which no one else can undergo for it. This learning process is nothing other than the 'I' acquiring capacities which it originally failed to develop consciously and which it must now accrue on a different level — no longer freely, but as a matter of necessity. As these inner processes occur during the course of the illness, the 'I' is enabled to reassess its situation (comprehension of destiny), overcome self-built obstacles (achieve independence), as well as assimilate initially unexpected external influences (coming to terms with destiny).

AIDS — a karmic benefit?

If the dual aspects of illness are ignored, illness is judged exclusively in negative terms as an accident or the result of the vagaries of nature, as a breakdown, etc. An attitude towards illness which accords with human dignity sees it as the intimate field of a person's experience in which the individual can progress in his development. As such, illness becomes an indispensable part of human existence.

AIDS is a truly terrible illness and we should not fail to do anything which might prevent it or help in its treatment. Yet, following the issues raised in this book, we may be allowed to ask whether there might be a 'karmic benefit'. We have already developed certain ideas and images with regard to both the conscious and the deeply unconscious experiences of the 'I' in the processes connected with acquired immunodeficiency.

In view of karma, we need to ask why an individual in the twentieth century 'seeks' experiences in which the physical correlate of the 'I' is destroyed, in which its organic basis is dissolved and deprived of any firm foundation. Are karmic illusions, far-reaching mistakes, corrected through experiences which occur in the course of the illness? This question may be tentatively answered if we look at human spiritual awareness throughout the last two thousand years. In still earlier millennia of human history the spiritual nature of human beings was a directly accessible fact.

The awareness of the spiritual nature of human beings has gradually faded. Increasingly, the consequence has been the tragic, historical confusion between body and self. But since the start of the modern era (15th century) this has been not only a mere theoretical confusion but how life in reality has been experienced. An initially theoretical materialism became practical materialism, which has influenced all spheres of life. The 'I' was mistaken for the body which it had formed.

This development is a particularly tragic one, because human beings require a body for their development on earth, but must not be seen as identical with it. Put another way, the spiritual element in human beings requires the sensory nature of the body in order to fulfil its task on earth, but as human beings we must not be seen as identical with the sensory nature of the body — otherwise we will fail to fulfil that task. The practice of materialism leads only to a 'pointless adherence to the senses' [102] in all areas of life. If the unique entity of the 'I' becomes identified with the body, whose origins lie in the species, the former becomes interchangeable and loses its identity.

But the confusion between spirit, soul and body, the loss of individuality, affects not only the relationship to one's own body but also to one's fellow human beings, particularly those of the opposite sex. If, in sexual relations, human beings fail to seek the spirit and the soul of the other person *through the medium* of the body, sexuality turns into the 'pointless adherence to the senses'. The latter can be recognized in a frequent change of sexual partners, indiscriminate promiscuity, in which relationships between human beings become nothing more than relationships between bodies. Such an environment is particularly conducive to AIDS.

We can understand that individuals whose karmic circumstances have led them into such a confusion of the 'I' with the body seek experiences in illness which correct this confusion — not only in theory, but in practice. For the experience of the deprivation of any firm foundation in the body will lead all the more strongly to the emergence of the autonomy of the spiritual individual, even if the illness is fatal. Living in his sick body, the AIDS patient can reverse, deep in his unconscious, the false identification with his body by experiencing: 'I am not my body; I am a spiritual being for whom my body only serves as an

---

[102] Rudolf Steiner, *The Deed of Christ and the Opposing Spiritual Powers*, Steiner Book Centre, Vancouver 1976, lecture of 22 March 1909.

instrument.' This experience provides a powerful force for the future — it is the karmic benefit of the illness.

Therapeutic aims — a perspective

Caring for AIDS patients means overcoming one's own fear. Help and care free of fear create the proper therapeutic atmosphere.

That does not mean carelessness and inattention when dealing with the infectious material from the patient. Such carelessness serves no purpose. Of what, then, can help and therapy consist, with an illness which at present appears incurable? It is self-evident that every form of prevention, whether through hygiene, vaccination or other forms of prophylaxis, occupies a significant position. The debate about the various ways of individual and social prevention does not belong within the framework of this book. This debate is in full swing and here, too, much still needs to be learnt about this completely new illness. The urgent necessity to give psychological support to patients has led to the establishment of numerous self-help groups and other advice centres. They are to be welcomed. But psychological help should be extended to take the spiritual aspects of the illness into account. A person who will certainly die as a result of his illness should have a knowledge of the spiritual independence of his individual self and of its continued existence beyond death. But he also needs the tools to grasp this individuality through his own experience. It is of greatest importance for the AIDS patient to raise into consciousness the deeply subconscious physical experience of the spiritual independence of his self in relation to his disappearing immune system. The first steps on the way to the patient's spiritual experience of his inner autonomy in relation to the body are also the first steps towards a 'cure', a correction of the karmically based false identification of body and 'I'.

The fight against the physical symptoms of AIDS has sparked off intensive medical research. 'Whoever sees into these things', Rudolf Steiner says in his discussion of the esoteric causes of infectious diseases, 'will, of course, not take them as a reason for opposing modern medicine with its external remedies. But a real improvement will never come about through these external methods.' [103]

The first medicines to affect the virus are being tested and are available on the market. It remains to be seen how they work. Therapeutic considerations should be included in this work which create a link with what we have discussed above. For we may ask how immunological recognition, immunological resistance of the unconscious 'I', the biological individual, can be strengthened through therapeutic forces in nature. [104]

AIDS is active on many levels. Therapy and prophylaxis must start on all of them. The spiritual life of modern society, and thus its moral life as a community of nations and as a world community, must be treated and healed on the basis of the underlying causes. AIDS is proving to be an indicator of the situation of civilized humanity, the touchstone of the twentieth century. If we succeed in making a proper assessment of this situation, both in understanding and action, and if we draw the consequences from that for a transformed civilization, then AIDS — still an incurable illness — will also be overcome.

---

[103] Rudolf Steiner, *Foundations of Esotericism*, lecture of 3 November 1905.
[104] Dr med. Bernardo Kaliks, 'Die AIDS-Krankheit und die Ich — Organisation des Menschen', in: *Beiträge zu einer Erweiterung der Heilkunst*, Vol. 40, No. 4, July/August 1987.